Sage Principles

Discourses on Tàijí Medicine

Sage Principles

Discourses on Tàijí Medicine

Cheng Man-ch'ing

Foreword by Barbara Davis

Translated by

Tam Gibbs, Ed Young & Stephen Cowan

Edited by Daniel Schrier

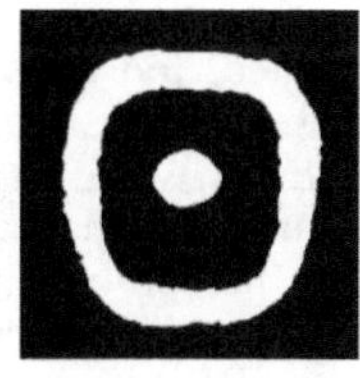

Ring Press Collective

Published by Ring Press Collective,
San Diego, CA & Cortlandt Manor, NY

ISBN - 979-8-9926868-2-1
First Edition Printing: March 2026
Library of Congress Control Number: 2026907474

Cover Artwork: Ed Young
Cover Design: Emily Do
Back Cover Photo: Ken Van Sickle
Book Editing, Layout and Design: Daniel Schrier

Disclaimer:

This book is designed to provide useful information on the subject matter covered and should not be considered a substitute for advice from a medical professional, whom the reader should consult before beginning any diet or exercise regime and before taking any Chinese herbal formulas, dietary supplements or other medications.

This text is sold with the understanding that this information is scholarly in nature and is in no way meant to be a practical hands-on guide to prescriptive medicine by non-Traditional Chinese Medicine (TCM) practitioners. All readers seeking such guidance are directed to seek professional education, including Chinese medical diagnosis techniques, which are not included in this text. As with any form of medicine, preventative or curative, herbal, chemical, ingested or performed, readers should NOT self-medicate or administer these treatments to others without appropriate education from licensed professionals. The author, publisher, and editor shall have neither liability nor responsibility to any person or entity with respect to any loss, injury, or damage caused, directly or indirectly, by the information contained in this book. It is imperative that you consult a licensed physician or other licensed healthcare provider before considering any of the measures discussed in this publication.

Dedication

To Professor Cheng for all he has passed on to us.

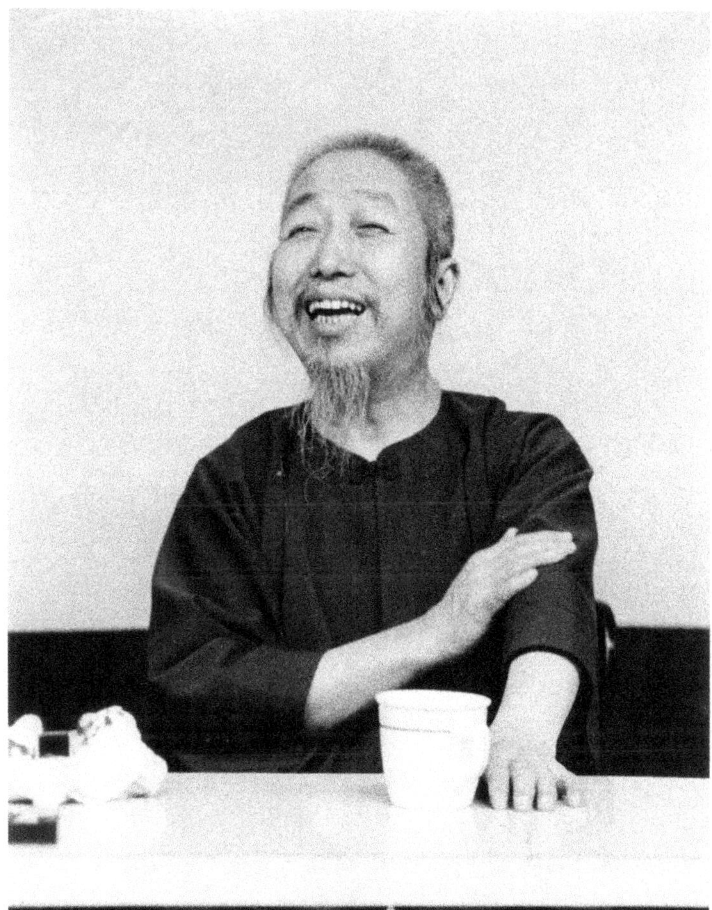

Cheng Man-ch'ing 郑曼青 (1902-1975)
Photo attributed to Ken Van Sickle

The Ring Press Collective:
Publisher's Mission Statement

Ring Press Collective was established to provide a platform for a collective group of East Asian Medicine practitioners who propose that the practice of "Ecological Medicine" is desperately needed in the 21st century world at large. Application of the principles of *yīnyáng* 陰陽, *wǔxíng* 五行 (five phases), channel theory, and seasonal *qì*, emphasize the importance of living in coherence with Change. Such change is governed by solar, lunar, sidereal, diurnal, seasonal and yearly cycles that inform and guide our practice of Chinese medicine in lifestyle as well as therapeutics. Our work encourages deep study and reflection on the classics, living in accordance with the processes of *Dào* 道, in order to reduce the current stresses on our planet caused by strains on resources, ecological damage, and loss of connection to heavenly and earthly *qì*. Our aim is to provide texts, media and resources that inspire our fellow human beings to walk with grace upon our planet, in harmony with all sentient beings. The clinical tools at our disposal include acupuncture/moxibustion, herbal medicine, counseling, dietetics, *qìgōng* 氣功, *tàijí* 太極, yoga, and meditation practices. We at *Ring Press Collective* wish to make these tools and texts available to as many people as possible, in order to build a better world and ensure a future for our children, grandchildren and beyond, while honoring the ecological, medical and philosophical teachings bestowed upon us by our ancestors.

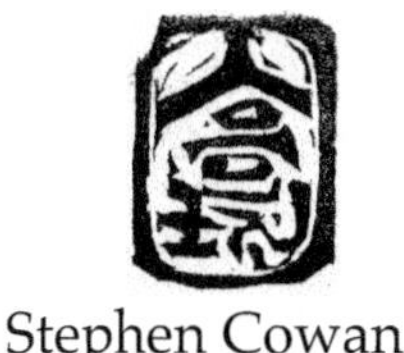
Stephen Cowan

Z'ev Rosenberg

Acknowledgements

"In the northern darkness there is a fish and his name is K'un. The K'un is so huge I don't know how many thousand li he measures. He changes and becomes a bird whose name is P'eng. The back of the P'eng measures I don't know how many thousand li across and, when he rises up and flies off, his wings are like clouds all over the sky. When the sea begins to move, this bird sets off for the southern darkness, which is the Lake of Heaven."

First lines of *Zhuāngzǐ* 《莊子》 Chapter One[1]
"Free and Easy Wandering."

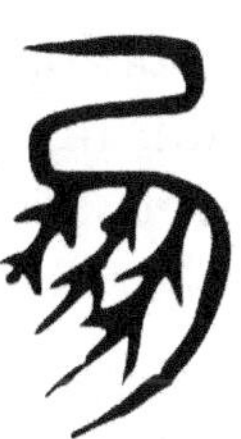

Like any long journey, there have been many friends and acquaintances who have helped bring this labor of love to fruition. Ed once said to me, in child-like awe, "I am surrounded by geniuses." At the time he was referring to a carpenter who had figured out a way to fix one of his cabinets. But he was also thinking about another friend who knew how to work his computer. The character for friend *péng* 朋 in modern Chinese looks like two moons but the ancient seal form (seen above) shows a large bird, *Péng*, similar to old Zhuāngzǐ's big bird. According to the *Shuōwén jiězì* 《说文解字》 (Han dynasty dictionary), the character depicts a flock of birds flying in formation, numbering in the tens of thousands;

hence it was used to represent a group of friends, flying in the same direction.

This book is such a bird given flight by the *tàijí* 太極 community and those friends of Ed's and mine who accompanied us, questioned us, encouraged us to stay the course. In particular, Cathy Chou, who opened our eyes to the 175 Characters, and Barbara Davis for her important contributions to the text. Deep bows to Ellyce Cavanaugh, who gave us constant moral support, as well as to the whole Sunday Vessel zoom group whose lively conversations added *qì*-breath to our free and easy wanderings: Will Morrison, Liam Comerford, Jean Zimmermann, Denny Sirotta, Natasha Gorky-Young, Mil Romanow, Carolyn Hoffman, Amelia Carling, Susan Heineman, Mark Westcott, George Chiang, Jano Cohen, Jim Depeyster, Laurie Seeman, David Janeway, Redmond Entwhistle, Richard Iannuzzi, Wendy Goulston, Barry Strugatz and to Peg Morris for her "eagle eye" during the very early and very late stage editing. Other wings in the flock include Patrick Cavanaugh and Djemila Lekouara, as well as Wolfe Lowenthal and the Long River *tàijí* camp, who allowed us to present some of this material one summer in Amherst. Additional support, inspiration and creativity provided by the brilliant Daniel Kelm, and Greta Sibley, Anita Soos and Sean Kernan, who all sat around on one stormy day in the North country to chew on the meaning and artistry of Professor's characters.

A special thanks to the Cheng family for giving Ed permission to bring this material that he's been carrying around for 50 years to the public. And to Antonia and Ananda Young, many thanks for their skill in sorting through Ed's many papers.

This book of course could never have taken flight without the tireless editing efforts and expertise of Daniel Schrier; the Dao is strong in him.

Finally, deep bows of gratitude to the spirit of the ancestor-sages who have been our constant companions on this long distance flight. May they continue to support Professor Cheng's words into the future.

[1] Watson, (1968). *The Complete Works of Chuang Tzu* p. 29.

Table of Contents

List of Figures and Illustrations

Zhèng Mànqīng's Medical Journey by Barbara Davis

The Lotus

Lifting itself above the earth,
not stained by the dirty mud;
Placed in a simple surrounding
unexpectedly nature's truth is revealed.
I paint the lotus flower,
but it laughs at me;
Its everlasting fragrance faces
a hundred-year-old mortal only for a moment.

— Zhèng Mànqīng 郑曼青, 1963[2]

Professor Zhèng Mànqīng (1902–1975) was known as a "Master of Five Excellences" for his talents in five fields: poetry, calligraphy, painting, *tàijí quán* 太極拳 (*t'ai-chi ch'üan*), and traditional Chinese medicine. To him, these arts were deeply interwoven in their theory and practice and in the ways they explored self and the world around. As he quoted Confucius, "My Dao is strung together as if on one thread."[3]

Zheng was born in Yǒngjiā 永嘉, Zhèjiāng 浙江 Province in southeastern China.[4] The sixth child, Zhèng was bright but sickly, and did not walk until he was several years old. The family faced a number of calamities, including the death of his father. They became impoverished, and moved in with Mrs. Zhèng's family, the Zhangs.[5] Zhèng Mànqīng's mother (1875–1960) was known for being skilled with herbs and took the young boy along on herb-gathering walks.[6] She also taught him calligraphy and chanted the great classics of poetry to him. Her younger sister, Zhāng Hóngwēi 張紅薇 (1878–1970), was a skilled artist who encouraged the young boy in painting and poetry since he was already showing artistic leanings.[7]

Around the age of nine, Zhèng Mànqīng was outside playing with friends, when suddenly, something fell from above and struck him on the head, knocking him unconscious for two days. He was revived with herbal remedies, however, his memory was gone. Aunt Hóngwēi's painting teacher, Wāng Xiāngchán 汪香禪 (1867–1923), took Zhèng as an assistant in his studio, having the boy grind ink and do simple tasks as he recovered his strength and memory.[8] As the boy continued to recuperate, he tried his own hand, painting on scraps of paper. One day, Teacher Wāng came across one of Zhèng's paintings and declared him ready to be a professional. As was the custom, Teacher Wang bestowed a studio name upon Zhèng—Wisteria—and set prices for his works.[9]

Adulthood

At about fourteen, Zhèng Mànqīng moved to nearby Hángzhōu 杭州, one of China's most important artistic locales. There he befriended artists and poets, studied more, and began to sell his paintings in order to help support his family. Around 1919, he moved to Běijīng 北京, where he obtained a position teaching poetry at Yuwen College.[10] Though he was only in his late teens, he became part of Běijīng's artistic circles.

As Zhèng Mànqīng came of age, the country was in profound upheaval: political and ideological battles, tradition and modernization, Western-influenced educational reforms, and pressures from foreign powers.

In the midst of all this, in the mid-1920s, Zhèng moved to Shanghai, the center of China's artistic world. He and Aunt Hongwei were featured participants in national and international exhibits, both lauded as "Masters of Three Excellences" (poetry, calligraphy, and painting).[11]

Changes were happening in the art world, as well, via the institutionalization of art education, promotion of overseas study, use of Western subjects and mediums, shifts in patronage, and opening of museums. Zhèng was hired to lead the department of traditional painting the prestigious Shanghai College of Art. In his new role, Zhèng brought on many of his well-known colleagues as faculty, and later, with painter Huáng Bīnhóng 黃賓虹 (1865–1955), founded the Chinese Cultural College, drawing instructors from this same circle of influential artists. Unfortunately, the school only operated briefly.

Traditional Medicine

Health care in China was undergoing the same radical changes as the art world, and was yet one more battleground over modernization and social reform. The medical establishment adopted Western medicine techniques with its focus on disease, hospitals, surgery, equipment, and science, rather than clinging to ancient Chinese theories of *qi*, balance, and harmony. These Chinese medical traditions had for thousands of years employed modalities such as herbs, acupuncture, massage, *qìgōng*, diet, poultices, and cupping, while practitioners could come from folk and family-lineages such as Zhèng's mother, itinerant healers who plied their skills from town to town, or scholar-physicians who used highly developed classical theories.

"Chinese medicine" was not a monolithic system. It consisted of many diverse styles of practice as well as regional variations, since diseases and remedies were intrinsically linked to local climate and geography. A southern practitioner would have expertise in Warm Diseases, but in the north, a practitioner would rely on "Cold Damage" theories. Whatever the theory, *prevention* was the goal, beginning with proper eating, sleeping, and activity, all to be in accord with the seasons and an individual's constitution.

Every medical system, though, has its gaps. In the case of Chinese medicine, it was weak in public health: opium addiction, malnourishment, and communicable diseases were rampant. Western medicine was stronger in that arena. In the mid-1800s, Christian missionaries had brought Western medicine—itself still developing—to China, where they established clinics and hospitals. Though their efforts were sometimes tinged with attitudes of cultural superiority, they helped fill some of the gaps in Chinese health care; cataract surgery being one of their biggest successes. (The opposite situation would later happen in 1960s America, when Chinese medicine, influenced in part by immigrants such as Zhèng Mànqīng, began to make inroads, offering "holistic" care that filled gaps within Western medicine.)

The dire health care challenges in early twentieth century China spurred Chinese government officials to endorse a turn away from the thousands of years of accumulated traditional knowledge in search of efficacious, scientific answers. Western medicine even made inroads in poorer and rural communities who could not afford traditional doctors or herbal treatments.

While in Shanghai, Zhèng Mànqīng suffered from overwork at the art school and was stricken with Lung disease (what Western medicine would likely call tuberculosis). He had become so ill that "he had been told he should go home and prepare to die. He went and bought medical books, figuring there was nothing left to lose by trying to treat himself."[12] He sampled herbs, and practiced on himself.

Zhèng's study of Chinese medicine was not necessarily unusual for someone of his intellect and temperament. For one thing, traditional medicine was one more means of being of service, lifting the spirits of a weakened country. Always an able autodidact, Zhèng studied the ancient medical classics, among them, the *Yellow Emperor's Inner Classic, Celestial Pivot,* and *Plain Questions,* later classics such as *Discussion of Cold Damage,* the herbal Materia Medica, prescriptions from the *Golden Chest,* and handy references such as those from the *Great Compendium of Acupuncture and Moxibustion.* These classics described theories and applications—from qi to nutrition to attacks of pernicious forces—that formed the bases of the many schools of Chinese medical theory. Hundreds of essays, diagrams, poems, and ditties catalogued the signs and symptoms of illnesses, herbal properties and prescriptions, and acupuncture point locations and functions. All of these would need to be memorized and integrated into one's practice.[13]

Word got around about Zhèng's medical knowledge and he began to write herbal prescriptions for friends. But although he had studied much on his own, there was no substitute for learning at the side of a master doctor. That way, one could receive the accumulated wisdom of a lineage and discuss real-life cases, which were inherently more complex than presented in a case book.

At one point, Zhèng visited a doctor with whom he thought he might study: *"After showing me a score of delicately illustrated books, he said that I would have to spend twelve years studying and never leave his side. I thanked him, and went to search for another teacher. As it turned out, I spent well over thirty years studying the basics of acupuncture."*[14]

Around 1926, Zhèng met a retired doctor of traditional medicine named Sòng Yòu'ān 宋幼庵, who lived in the mountains in Anhui province, about 200 miles west of Shanghai.[15] Sòng was a ninth-generation doctor in his seventies. Apparently Sòng's own four sons—all said to be famous doctors—did not have the temperament or interest necessary for carrying on the "mysteries" of the family tradition.[16]

How Sòng and Zhèng met was a bit of a comedy of errors. Dr. Sòng happened to have come to Shanghai to meet with an old friend. Someone showed him a prescription that Zhèng had written. Sòng assumed, given the prescription's subtlety, that the doctor who wrote it was an older, experienced practitioner. Sòng stopped by Zhèng Mànqīng's college in Shanghai and left him a note. But Zhèng was wrapped up with school obligations. Sòng came three times, each time leaving a note.

They finally met, and Zhèng was eager to study with Sòng and wanted to *kowtow* to Sòng, but Sòng wanted to teach him regardless of their age differences. They finally came to an agreement, that Zhèng would instead bow to Sòng's ancestors. It was unusual for Sòng to search out someone outside of his own family, or for that matter, for a master to search out a student; normally, a student would seek the master, through an introduction. However, Sòng was drawn to this young man who exhibited the traits Sòng sought, someone "who was smart, of good character, who would not view medicine as a skill with which just to become rich, but rather to help people."[17]

Since Zhèng still had a heavy load of responsibilities at school, he was only able to go study for two summers with Sòng.[18] When Zhèng would come, Sòng would place ads in the newspaper to drum up clientele who had serious illnesses.[19] In this way, Zhèng learned to treat the most challenging cases. In the case of certain contagious diseases, Sòng advised Zhèng to have a drink of liquor prior to seeing the patient, as it would "raise his qi" to help prevent him catching their illness.[20]

After his studies with Song, Zhèng hung out his shingle, and soon earned the nickname "One-dose Zhèng" for the efficacy of his prescriptions, some of which were carried by pharmacies and advertised in the newspaper.[21] Zhèng later wrote several tracts on traditional herbal medicine, and became involved with national politics by becoming a legislative representative of the traditional doctors.

Tàijí Quán Study

Zhèng found another important aid for healing his own illness: *tàijí quán*, which was yet one more way to study balance and movement of qi. At that time, martial arts such as *tàijí quán* played an important role in the national "self-strengthening" movement, and was popular among the scholarly class.

Zhèng had learned a bit of *tàijí quán* and qigong earlier, but now took it up seriously, gaining entrance to study with the famed Yáng Chéngfǔ 杨澄甫 (1883–1936). With his medical training, Zhèng helped Yáng's wife recover from a serious illness; Yáng then held nothing back in teaching him *tàijí quán*.

Zhèng created a "short form" of *tàijí quán*—thirty-seven moves total—in hopes of spreading it further. In the 1940s, Zhèng wrote his influential *Zhengzi's Thirteen Treatises on Tàijí Quán*.[22] In this book, Zhèng discussed *tàijí quán* practice and its benefits from philosophical, health, and practical points of view, including a full chapter covering Lung disease, his own experiences, the importance of mental attitude, the causes of illness, and the use of *tàijí quán* for recovery.

Changes

Zhèng married Dīng Wéizhuāng 丁惟莊 (Ting Wei-chuang; 1916–2005), an obstetrician, in 1941, and began a family that would ultimately have three daughters and two sons. Wartime pressures forced them to move west to Chongqing, Zhèng put his medical skills to use during the Sino-Japanese war, when he and his wife and Aunt Hóngwēi 紅薇 lived in Chongqing, Sichuan Province. During this time, Zhèng also served as a medical advisor to Generalissimo Chiang Kai-shek 蔣介石 (1887–1975), the leader of the Republic of China government.

After relocating to Taiwan at the end of the civil war in 1949, Zhèng set up his medical practice in the living room of their home. There he would receive patients, read their pulses, and write out prescriptions to be filled at a nearby pharmacy. He would often adjust fees for people in need, or, after the person left, would call ahead to the pharmacy and tell them to put the herbs on his own tab.[23]

Zhèng kept a busy schedule, participating in the legislature, and supporting the Cultural Renaissance Movement. His interest in art and poetry continued; with a half-dozen art colleagues he created the "Seven Friends of Painting," who held frequent joint exhibits, and he also formed a poetry group. During this time, Zhèng also served as a painting tutor to Chiang Kai-chek's wife Sòng Měilíng 宋美齡 (1898-2003).

In late 1963, Zhèng Mànqīng and his wife visited Europe, where he had a one-man painting exhibit at the prestigious Museé Cernuschi in Paris. After New Year's, they stopped in New York City for a lengthy visit. They decided to resettle there, ultimately bringing their five children, now in their teens and twenties, from Taiwan, taking an apartment on the Upper West Side of Manhattan.

Zhèng began teaching *tàijí quán* in New York, initially at his host Da Liu's apartment, and then at the New York T'ai Chi Ch'uan Association at 211 Canal Street in Chinatown, a group organized by local businessmen. Word got around about the classes, and soon there was an influx of outsiders; in this way Zhèng became one of the first Chinese *tàijí quán* masters to teach openly in the US and to regularly take on non-Chinese students. At the studio, he also saw patients, and sent them with their prescriptions to the local herbal pharmacies. In 1971, Zhèng and numerous students relocated and formed the Shr Jung Association, which met at 87 Bowery in Manhattan.

The 1960s and 1970s in the United States was for Americans a time of great curiosity about Eastern teachings. Chinese medicine was at that time virtually unknown outside of the Chinatowns of larger American cities. Any practice was done sub rosa and was hard to find; outsiders coming into an herbal pharmacy would be viewed with suspicion. It would be another decade before there was any real awareness of Chinese medicine, let alone regulation.

A steady flow of patients came to consult Zhèng Mànqīng. Some were students, others came by word-of-mouth. They had a range of problems from general aches and pains, infertility, venereal disease, to extremely complex ones, including a young autistic boy. For the most part, Zhèng practiced herbs, though he always travelled with a kit of needles, as it was good to be prepared for emergencies.[24]

Zhèng was keen on imparting the health-enhancing ideas and practices of China, particularly as he was encountering so many non-Chinese students who had little or no exposure to these ideas, and many of whom were in search of stability. Because of this, he commenced giving numerous lectures to the New York students about Confucius (Kǒngzǐ 孔子), Lǎozǐ 老子, the Doctrine of the Mean (*Zhōngyōng* 《中庸》), and healthful living. Zhèng used every opportunity to educate his students about leading healthier lives. *Tàijí quán* practice was of great importance, but he saw much else that needed attention: diet, sleep, and proper sexual conduct. The latter drew much of his attention, since this was a time in the United States of drastic change of sexual mores, so much so that Zhèng made note of a patient he saw who did *not* have venereal disease.[25]

Zhèng Mànqīng spent his last eleven years between New York City and Taibei, teaching *tàijí quán*, giving herbal consultations, writing, painting, and exhibiting his art. Zhèng wrote at least a dozen books during this period—on poetry, philosophical essays, commentaries on classics, *tàijí quán*, medicine, and the arts.

Connections between Zhèng's various arts abounded: the sensitivity and finger dexterity required for acupuncture needling and massage techniques were no different than an artist's handling of ink, brush, and paper, or a *tàijí quán* player's touch in sword or push hands. The careful balance of elements in a painting was equivalent to the construction of an herbal formula. In Zhèng's hands, all of these arts were vehicles for the study of the Dao.

Zhèng passed away in 1975 at seventy-three, while on an extended visit to Taiwan, leaving behind family and thousands of students. He may be known best for his *tàijí quán*; however, he had a quieter role in helping preserve traditional Chinese medicine and bring it to a new realm, as numbers of his students, and in turn, their students helped establish Chinese medicine in the West. Above all, he transmitted the ideals of ancient China to new generations and cultures.

Barbara Davis, M.A.
Director, Cheng Man-ch'ing Biography Project
https://chengmanching.wordpress.com

Zhèng Mànqīng writings about Chinese Medicine:

- *Eight Important Points On Cancer* (*Tan ai bayao*), 1966. Pamphlet. Excerpts translated in *Master of Five Excellences*, Hennessy, 1995 (North Atlantic Books / Frog).
- *Essence of Gynecology* (*Nuke xinfa*). 1961. Trans. Wile, 2011 (Sweet Ch'i Press), and excerpts translated in *Master of Five Excellences*, Hennessy, 1995 (North Atlantic Books / Frog).
- Subtleties of Orthopedics (Guke jingwei). Not extant.

Foreword Notes:

---

[2] Translated by Dr. S. D. Ren from the *Shr Jung* Anniversary Booklet.

[3] Analects of Confucius, 4.15.1.

[4] Yǒngjiā 永嘉 (Yung-chia) is now known as Wēnzhōu 溫州. Below, ages are approximate within one or two years and given according to Western customs. Names are given surname first. Pinyin romanization is used, supplemented with Wade-Giles in parentheses. The bulk of biographical information in this introduction is drawn from Tam Gibbs, "*Cheng Tzu: Master of the Five Excellences*" in *Full Circle*, vol. 1 no. 2 (June 1985, pp. 13–21), unless otherwise indicated. Gibbs' article has a prefatory note, "November 2, 1978. This translation was done in the presence of Mrs. Cheng as she transliterated the *wenyan* [classical Chinese] of Professor Cheng's funerary book into *baihua* [vernacular] so that I could understand it.

Zhèng's names are as follows (pinyin followed by Wade-Giles, pronunciation, and meaning). His given name: Yuè 岳/Yüeh/*you-eh* "Mountain Peak"; courtesy name: Mànqīng/Man-ch'ing/*mahn ching* 曼青 "Luxuriantly Green"; assumed name in 1950s: Mànrán 曼髯/Man-jan/*mahn rahn* "Luxuriant Whiskers." He also used artistic monikers, in particular, *Yùjǐng shān rén* 玉井山人/Yu-ching shan-jen "Hermit of the Jade Well"; and (*Liánfù* 蓮父/Lien-fu), "Father of the Lotus." Note that a person can use a number of names or nicknames, depending on their stage of life or context.

[5] Zhèng's mother and father's names are not known, and both surnames are quite common. Her family name is Zhāng 張 (Chang, pronounced jahng).

[6] Her dates are mentioned in Zhèng's preface to *Renwen qianshuo*, p. i.

[7] Zhāng Hóngwēi 張红薇 (Chang Hung-wei) became a well-known artist and art educator who painted in the "birds and flowers" genre.

[8] Wāng Xiāngchán 汪香禪 (Wang Hsiang-ch'an) was from Longxiang, Zhejiang Province. He had over thirty students, a number of whom became well-known painters and calligraphers. "*Liushi nian lai xi hua suo tan*" (Chatting About the Past Sixty Years of Painting), p. 14, in *Yi tan*, 39/6 (1971), pp. 14–24.

[9] According to Yao Menggu's bio from funerary book, the name is *téng huā guǎn* 藤花館 (*téng* 藤 is rattan, cane, and also written 籐 (bamboo on top) Generically climbing vines such as wisteria.

[10] No further information has been found about this school.

[11] See Jane Zheng's *The Modernization of Chinese Art: The Shanghai Art College, 1913-1937*. Leuven, Belgium: Leuven University Press, 2016; and Pedith Chan *The Making of a Modern Art World: Institutionalisation and Legitimisation of Guohua in Republican Shanghai.* Boston: Brill, 2017

[12] Wayne and Patrick Cheng interviews, August 2006.

[13] For more on Chinese medicine, see Dominique Hoizey, *A History of Chinese Medicine* (Edinburgh University Press, 1993, and Paul Unschuld, *Medicine in China: A History of Ideas* (University of California Press, 1988).

[14] Article from China Post or China News, c. 1974. "Arts Master Triumphs Over All." This mention of "acupuncture" was possibly meant as a generic reference to traditional Chinese medicine, a common catch-all term in the United States, as acupuncture was initially the most visible and "exotic" modality practiced; in China, herbal remedies often predominate.

[15] Additional information on Zheng's studies with Sòng Yòu'ān 宋幼庵 (Sung You-an) is drawn from interviews with Zheng's children (9/28/06), Mrs. Cheng (interviewed by Epi Van Pol, 2004). No further information has been found about Sòng in standard medical references; however, Sòng is a common surname, and it is possible that he was known by a different personal name.

[16] It may have been that Sòng's sons had become doctors of *Western* medicine; thus Song might have turned to someone outside the family.

[17] Patrick Cheng interview, 3/8/06

[18] Katy and Wayne Cheng interviews, August 2006.

[19] It was common for newspapers to carry ads for medicines and practitioners.

[20] Katy and Wayne Cheng interview, August 2006.

[21] During the 1930s, Zhèng also studied literature and writing for several years with the retired scholar Qián Míngshān 錢名山 (c. 1875–1944, Ch'ien Ming-shan).

[22] *Zhèng zǐ tàijí quán shísān piān* 郑子太极拳十三篇 (*Thirteen Treatises*, 1950).

[23] Wayne and Patrick Cheng interview, August 2006.

[24] Wayne Cheng, interview, 2006.

[25] Wolfe Lowenthal, *There Are No Secrets: Professor Cheng Man-ch'ing's T'ai Chi Ch'uan.* Berkeley: North Atlantic Books, 1991, p. 13.

Preface by Cheng Man-ch'ing 郑曼青

The "Sage Principles" (*zhéli* 哲理)[26] of China embrace the three dimensions of Heaven, Earth and Human. Their meanings are so profound that people discussing them in the last hundred-odd years, both Chinese and Westerners alike, have not even reached a superficial understanding of what they really mean. The cause of this is that most interpretations of the *Yìjīng* 《易經》 (*Book of Changes*)[27] and the *Lǎozi* 《老子》[28] relied on Wáng Bì 王弼's commentaries.[29] Wáng Bì's commentary was full of mistakes, which have caused considerable misunderstanding.

In this book, I have selected one hundred and seventy-five characters from the sayings of the ancient Chinese sages, such as the *Yìjīng* 《易經》 *(Book of Changes)* and its commentary by Confucius (Kǒngzǐ 孔子), *Huángdì nèijīng* 《黃帝內經》 (Emperor Huáng's *Internal Medicine Classic),* as well as Lǎozǐ's *Dàodé jīng* 《道德經》, which have an intimate relationship to *Tàijí quán* 太極拳 (*T'ai-chi ch'üan*) movements, and are based on a way of life which is in harmony with the principles of physiology and science.[30]

Chinese physiology is mainly based on a single work: Emperor Huáng's *Internal Medicine Classic.* Its principle is so thorough and profound that one studying it must exercise utmost patience and must consistently assume an objective attitude in order to achieve a complete understanding of its true meaning.

I will explain the meaning of those terms which have no equivalents in Western language and interpret the original sayings in detail in order to assist students studying *The Sage Principles* to reach understanding more easily.

With a faith that moves mountains, I will not rest until the goal is reached. It would be a satisfaction to me if, out of ten thousand readers, one or two could comprehend the true meaning of this text.

Cheng Man-ch'ing 郑曼青
From the town of Wen Chou 溫州
In Chekiang province 浙江省,
Written in New York City,
Winter 1966-67

Preface Notes:

---

26 *Zhéli* 哲理 (Sage Principles) - see Chapter One

27 *Yìjīng* 《易經》 (*Book of Changes; I-Ching*)

28 Usually known and referred to by its honorific title *Dàodé Jīng* 《道德經》 (*Scripture on the Dào and Inner Power; Lao-tzu)*

29 Wáng Bì 王弼 (Wang Pi) (226-249 CE) was an influential Chinese philosopher and neo-Daoist (*xuánxué* 玄學) scholar. He produced highly influential commentaries on the *Dàodé jīng* 《道德經》 and *Yìjīng* 《易經》 that helped shape their interpretation for centuries. Wáng Bì emphasized metaphysical principles such as *wú* 無 (non-being) as the generative ground of *yǒu* 有 (being), arguing that Daoist thought provided the philosophical foundation underlying Confucian ethics and social order.

---

30 Physiology (*shēnglǐ* 生理) is composed of two characters. *Shēng* 生 (birth, or life) and *lǐ* 理 (inner pattern,"reason, logic,"science). Scientific (*kēxué* 科学) the characters Professor Cheng is using for "science" is interesting: *kē* 科 means "department of science" and *xué* 学 means "learning" or "knowledge." Together they imply the area of scientific knowledge or scientific study. It is also important to remember that in this context *lǐ* 理 (principle, "reason,"internal pattern), is also translated as "science' in colloquial parlance. See Appendix III: *Etymological Glossary of Sage Principle Terms,* for a more detailed analysis of these characters.

Preface by Ed Young

Everything achieved in my life that amounts to anything worthwhile in human terms has been a byproduct of some other pursuits. For instance, I came to the U.S. to study architecture, shifted into advertising within three years, studied industrial design for another year and ended up as an author and illustrator of children's picture books for the past fifty years.

Also, in another realm, I suffered a severe knee injury in college. It worsened until I found a cure by an old Chinese physician and *tàijí* 太極 master, Professor Cheng Man-ch'ing, and ended up teaching with him and carrying on this teaching for the next fifty years.

Since I spoke English and Professor Cheng's native Chinese language, I was selected as one of his two translators (along with Tam Gibbs) during his presence in the US. By profession, I am a storyteller, and therefore able to serve menial translation needs in daily life. During those years, I witnessed countless patients brought back to health from "incurable" conditions as defined by Western medical doctors.

By 1975, Professor Cheng had been focused on writing his commentary on the *Yìjīng* 《易經》 (*Book of Changes*). It was during this time that he decided to write an introduction to the principles of healing with hopes of adding to the current Western medical practices and thereby promote health. It was during his trip to Taiwan with the intention of publishing his *Yìjīng* commentary that he unexpectedly passed away. The unfinished manuscript remained first in Tam Gibb's possession and then was passed to me when he died. Though I understood that Professor Cheng left it for us with the intention of publishing in English, I was not able to take on the translation until I was in my sixties, thirty eight years later. While downsizing, the book resurfaced and I showed it to one of my long time *tàijí* students, Stephen Cowan, a medical doctor who had also studied Chinese medicine. Steve enthusiastically took an interest and offered to help me get this book into a form that could be printed. During the intervening years since Professor Cheng left us, I had also been studying the etymology of Chinese characters because of the deeper meanings hidden within the ideograms. It was then that Steve and I discovered the daunting task we must face as translators to cross the bridge between two entirely different cultures which share no identical words to communicate their unique perspectives. In other words, a Sinologist must find a word or phrase similar enough to express the ideas and concepts that are absent from Western culture to make do. This "make do" process then has been passed down through the ages as the "classics" of the original language. I began to ask, is this manner of passing on wisdom with all the best intention, truly a service to humanity then? No, not really, if anything, it runs the risk of being a disservice. Then does it mean no one should ever attempt to translate the thoughts and writings of another? My conclusion is "Yes, translations should be attempted," provided that the translator is part of the process by making the original available for further insight.

During the forty years since translating for Professor Cheng, I myself have been unhappy with the inadequacy of scholarly interpretations of Chinese culture and translations of characters into English. Although I have never thought of myself as a scholar of Chinese language (nor for that matter, do I think of myself as a scholar of any language, or any of the Chinese arts or classics), I do consider myself relatively proficient in *tàijí quán* 太極拳 and I have, as an artist, held a deep interest in the hidden meanings of Chinese symbols, having come to a place in my own life where I feel the necessity to unveil the mystery between the East-West, antiquity and modern myths revealed here in Professor Cheng's writings. In the ten years since we first undertook this painstaking translation, we have learned so much more of the medical knowledge that otherwise would have been missed in earlier versions of Professor's text. I can confidently say that what we introduce in this book with our interpretations of his words will enrich those students now and later to come, as well as demystifying the notion that East and West can never meet, because Professor Cheng certainly believed that there is such a place where the two meet, if you are open enough to let it.

May this bring some enlightenment to scholars in future generations. Perhaps, I venture to guess, this is yet another byproduct of my life's pursuits into unknown territory.

Ed Young
Cheng Man-ch'ing's interpreter,
Hastings-on-Hudson, NY
November 3, 2014
Year of the Wood Horse

Preface by Stephen Cowan, MD

During the late 1960's, Professor Cheng Man-ch'ing wrote this book at a time when there were no Western translations of Chinese medical texts available to the public. Today, the language and principles of Chinese medicine have become more familiar to Westerners and so Ed Young, who has been holding on to this text for over fifty years, felt the time might be right to share Professor's thoughts on health and medicine. As one of Ed's *tàijí* 太極 students, I was humbled and delighted to be asked to participate in the translation and preparation of Cheng Man-ch'ing's medical treatise entitled *Sage Principles.* My own practice of medicine was to be utterly transformed when I was first introduced to Chinese medicine in the early 1990s, and the medical classics have been an ongoing part of my study since that time.

Ed's commitment to honoring his teacher is unquestionable. The careful process with which he and I studied each character and phrase of Professor Cheng's writing in an attempt to accurately express the depth of his meaning has taken over fifteen years. This process has been a deeply meaningful learning experience for me personally as it has given me invaluable time with Ed, whose natural affinity as an artist for exploring Chinese ideograms brings out the multilayered meanings of the Professor's words.

Professor Cheng Man-ch'ing presents a vision of "*tàijí* medicine" as a holistic system of health, deeply grounded in the Confucian, Daoist and early medical classics. In so doing we get a glimpse of Professor Cheng as a role model of the sage-doctor who observes without bias, listens to what others can't hear, inquires with a compassionate heart and touches with what is known as "listening hands." As the master of five excellences: poetry (*shī* 詩), painting (*huà* 畫), *tàijí* 太極, calligraphy (*shū* 書) and medicine (*yī* 醫), Professor Cheng embodies the commitment to a natural ecological perspective and practice that respects the inseparability of mind-body-spirit thoroughly integrated into the rhythms of Nature. He approaches treating a patient the same way he paints a mountain stream or plays *tàijí*. This cultivation is a profound way of living that, for me, has been truly worth aspiring to.

In carefully examining the text of Professor's manuscript, it is clear to me how much he genuinely wished for Western medical practitioners to open their minds to the Chinese perspective of health. Chinese medicine is a complete system of medicine that does not fit so conveniently into the Western model of bio-reductionist theory. Indeed, Professor Cheng emphasizes this distinction from the very first chapter by differentiating the term "Sage Principles" from the Socratic "philosophies" that are the foundation of Western thought. His genuine hopes were that Western physicians might discover, through the Chinese sages, ways to deepen their spiritual commitment to their patients and thus provide more effective treatment.

At the time of writing this book, Professor Cheng was in the midst of completing his commentaries on the *Yìjīng* 《易經》 (*Book of Changes*), which clearly had a profound influence on his views of medicine. With emphasis on dynamic relations rather than fixed notions of static forms, Professor Cheng encourages us to think with a process-mindset that promotes our human growth potential.

The thirteen chapters of the *Sage Principles* are divided into two parts. The first seven chapters deal with the "high concepts" of the Chinese classics that describe the dynamic functions found in Nature while the second part of the book focuses on particular comparisons between Western and Chinese views of the human body. Throughout this book we can sense Professor's keen interest in, and curiosity about, the current scientific knowledge of Western medicine. We can imagine him turning the pages of *Cunningham's Textbook of Anatomy*, which he was apparently given at the time by one of his western medically-trained colleagues, and we get a rare opportunity to see how he interprets the anatomic illustrations through the eyes of a Chinese medical sage. According to Ed, the Professor wished to include a few of Cunningham's illustrations in the text. In so doing he applies the Sage principles such as the five-phase relations to our understanding of Heart disease (Ch. 8), the "*Tàijí* Principle" observed in a child's skeletal X-ray (Ch. 10) and the "microcosmic orbit (water wheel (*héchē* 河車) in understanding hormone function as a unified system (Ch. 13). These insights may challenge Western medical beliefs, but Professor Cheng does so without arrogance. Rather, he humbly offers us a glimpse of the "Sage Principles" in action, with a genuine spirit of hope that his vision of *tàijí* medicine will improve the health of our modern society.

My teacher and dear friend, Ed Young, passed away in 2023. He is sorely missed by all of us in the greater *tàijí* community.

I made a promise to Ed to complete the work on *Sage Principles* that he entrusted me with and to have it published in order to share Professor's thoughts with the world. This project has been a labor of love for both of us, yet we have been keenly aware that all translation is an ongoing interpretation linked to the context in which it is given life. Professor's texts were originally translated into English by Tam Gibbs and Ed at the time they were written in 1967. Ed and I began retranslating the text based on more accurate Chinese medical knowledge that hadn't been available to them when it was first encountered. Recognizing that the meaning of words and ideas is organic and will naturally change with time and with the particular perspectives of the reader, we have hoped that the *Sage Principles* and teachings will create new opportunities for dialogue that will continually give life to Professor Cheng's words.

It is with this intention that I humbly present this book.

Stephen Cowan MD
Year of the Fire Horse 2026

Cheng Man-ch'ing's Introduction

Explanation of Yīn-Yáng 陰陽 & the Five Phases (*Wúxíng* 五行)

I regard *yīn-yáng* 陰陽 and the five phases (*wúxíng* 五行) as the focal difference between Chinese and Western perspectives in particular as they relate to sage principles and Western science. The "Sage Principles" of China use *yīn-yáng* and the five phases as a bridge between philosophy and science whereas the lack of such a bridge in the West has resulted in their being considered separate domains of study. Here is my explanation:

The *yīn-yáng* principle lays out the intimate relationship between the Heavens (*yáng* 陽) and Earth (*yīn* 陰), likewise: male and female, hard and soft, hot and cold, dry and wet. All things have their *yīn* and *yáng* representations much like the symbolic factors x,y,z, used in algebra equations. The understanding that philosophy and science are manifestations of one principle is especially important in the field of medicine. For instance, in our time, both electrical and nuclear sciences can be reduced down to their lowest denominator of positive and negative charges, yet we still see the existence of two polar opposites. *Yīn-yáng* on the other hand, represent the alternating interrelationship of positive and negative poles in their mutual attraction and repulsion.

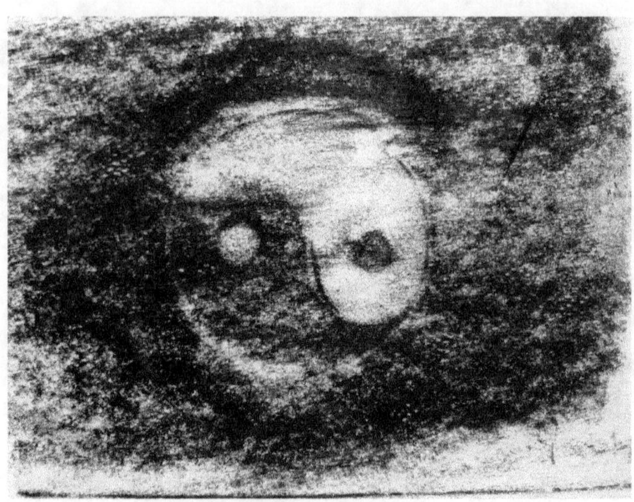

Figure 1: Tàijí Symbol
Rubbing created by Stephen Cowan and Ed Young

The imagery of the *yīn* (black circle) and *yáng* (white circle) as seen above in Figure 1, is traditionally traced to the legendary figure Fúxī 伏羲, who is said to have formulated the *Yìjīng's* 《易經》 eight trigrams (*bāguà* 八卦) over five millennia ago, in accordance with two ancient astrological diagrams: the *Hétú* 《河圖》 (*River Diagram*) and the *Luòshū* 《洛書》 (*Book of Lo*).[31] Confucius' commentary on the *Yìjīng* explains the *River Diagram* and the *Book of Lo* as corresponding to the great sages' concept of the five phases (*wǔxíng* 五行): Wood (*mù* 木), Fire (*huǒ* 火), Earth (*tǔ* 土), Metal (*jīn* 金), and Water (*shuǐ* 水), which have their mutual creative (*shēng* 生) and destructive (*kè* 克) relationships. According to the *Book of Lo*, the principle of the Heavens gives birth to Water and Earth gives birth to Fire. The *Yìjīng* employs the five phases to aid our understanding of the dynamic inter-relationships of *yīn-yáng* in a somewhat similar way that algebra employs numerical and alphabetical symbols to describe mathematical relationships.[32] For the sages however, these terms are not just abstract philosophical concepts; they do not separate form (*tǐ* 體) and function (*yòng* 用) in such a way that this unity actually supports today's scientific discoveries. The advances of modern science reflect the principles set down in China's past. This discussion is only suggested to show the wonder of the substance. One must still need to study further in order to attain its meaning.

Cheng Man-ch'ing

Introduction Notes:

---

31 *Luòshū* 《洛書》 (The *Book of Lo*) is a numerical diagram arranged in nine squares known as "the magic square" because the numbers add up to 15 in each direction (see Figure 4). This was considered the basis of the eight trigrams as will be explained in Chapter 3.

32 Professor Cheng implies here that certain Chinese symbols are employed in a similar way that numbers and mathematical symbols are used to represent larger concepts. These concepts will be explained in following chapters.

PART I

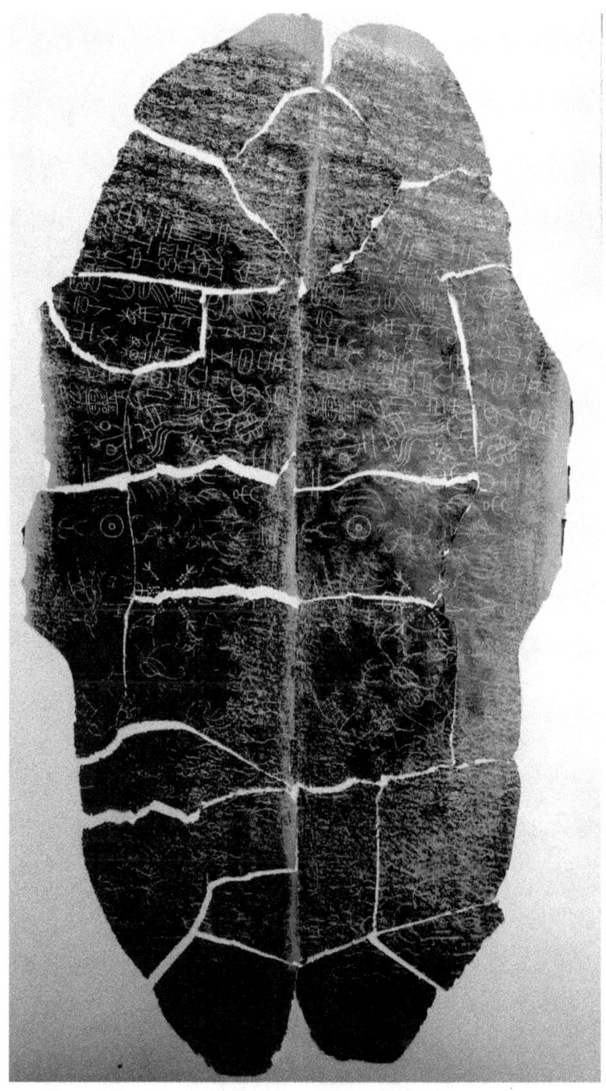

The 175 Sage Characters as if Written on a Turtle Shell
created by Ed Young

Chapter 1: The Sage Principles

Sage Teachings versus Philosophy

The translation of "Sage Teachings" (*zhéxué* 哲學) as "philosophy" should be corrected. The Chinese call their ancient Emperor Huang, (Huángdì 黃帝) "the Saint of Sages" (*shèngzhé* 聖哲). *The Book of History*[33] tells us that Emperors Yáo 堯 and Shùn 舜 developed the "Sage Civilization" (*zhé wén míng* 哲文明). Confucius (Kǒngzǐ 孔子, 551-479 BCE) called himself "Sage Man," (*shèngrén* 聖人) but later generations in China have never regarded him as having established a cult or school of "Sage Man teachings." This is in contrast to Socrates who, having expounded his "philosophy," was regarded as having established the "Socratic School."

The English translation of *zhéxué* 哲學[34] as "philosophy" rather than "sage teachings" is worth closer examination.[35] I find that the meaning of "philosophy" is very broad. Briefly stated, it is the love of knowledge and seeking of truth, branching out to all spheres of study. Excepting perhaps physiology and religion, it embraces the principles and systems of everything in the world and the entire cosmos. Accordingly, it seeks to undertake thorough research into the nature of truth by means of critical analysis. In effect, philosophy is really a body of literature that follows the reductive scientific method. If it were translated into Chinese, it would be more appropriate to call it the "study of intelligence," and its followers would be said to belong to different branches of intellectual study. Thus, if the Chinese term *zhéxué* or "sage teachings" were translated as philosophy, it would be like trying to put a square peg into a round hole: it just would not fit. Let me explain briefly the meaning of "Sage Principles and Teachings."

1. Emperor Huáng 黃, was called "Saint of Sages." His teaching, together with Lǎozi 老子's "Dào Principle" were known as "Sage Principles of Huáng Lǎo"[36] which expounds the principle of *wúwéi* 無為 (acting naturally or non-coercive action).
2. Emperor Yáo's 堯 and Emperor Shùn 舜's "Sage Civilization" was explained in the *Book of Changes* thus: "*Emperor Huáng, Yáo and Shùn ruled the empire by simply letting their robes hang gracefully.*"[37] This is to say that Emperors Yáo and Shùn inherited from Emperor Huáng the principle of "acting naturally" (*wúwéi* 無為).
3. Confucius (*Kǒngzǐ* 孔子; 551-479 BCE) called himself "Sage Man" (*zhérén* 哲人). His disciples praised him by calling him "Saint from Heaven."[38] They also addressed him as "Saint-Master."[39] To this Confucius humbly replied, "*As yet, a saint, I cannot be.*" By contrast, it appears that "saint" (*shèng* 聖) and "sage" (*zhé* 哲) can be considered in the same light as the difference between the Way (*Dào* 道) and its Virtues (*Dé* 德). The Way is given a name, just as "saint" is, while "virtues" (moral integrity) describe the effects or actions, just as "sage" does. Confucius did not want to be called "saint" because he already possessed the humility and substance of a "sage." From this it can be seen that the difference between "saint" and "sage" is similar to the difference between name and substance.

However, Confucius established the principles of human behavior by stating that in order to attain *Rén* 仁 (humaneness, benevolence, kindness, or universal love) and *Yì* 義 (justice, righteousness, or right conduct) one must use *kè qì* 客氣 (courtesy, modesty, or politeness) as the basis, and *zhōng yōng* 中庸 ("Middle Way," or "*Doctrine of the Mean*")[40] as the method of cultivating self-development, family harmony, tranquility of the nation and peace in the world. This begins by loving the "nine generations;" the four proceeding, the four following, and your own generation, and then extending your love to all people in general. Lǎozi 老子, on the other hand, has a different perspective. He says: "*I have the mind of a fool. To abandon education and discard intellect is my method.*"[41]

These then are the Chinese "Sage Principles" (*zhé lǐ* 哲理), which are very simple and clear, unlike Western "philosophy," which is broad and complex. As Confucius said: "*Why so many (schools of thought)? A mature person does not emphasize quantity.*"[42] If it is our purpose to build a bridge between Chinese and Western cultures, we must begin, as Confucius says, by defining the terms properly.[43] That's why it is necessary to explain the Chinese *zhé lǐ* 哲理 or "Sage Principles," as such, which should not be regarded as the same as the Western concept of philosophy.

Ch. 1 Notes

---

[33] *Shàng shūjīng* 《尚書經》 (*The Book of History*) one of the Five Classics of Confucius, was a collection of documents making up the oldest extant texts of Chinese history, from legendary times down to the times of Confucius.

---

34 In modern Chinese and Japanese dictionaries, *zhéxué* 哲學 is commonly translated as philosophy or philosophical teachings. See Appendix III: *Etymological Glossary of Sage Principle Terms*, for a more detailed analysis of the terms *zhé* 哲 (sage), *lǐ* 理 (principle) and *xué* 學 (teaching).

35 There is a subtle but important distinction between *zhé* 哲 and *shèng* 聖 worth noting. Both terms are often translated into English as "sage," though they carry different connotations in classical Chinese thought. See Appendix III: *Etymological Glossary of Sage Principle Terms*, for a more detailed analysis of these characters.

36 *Huáng Lǎo Zhé Lǐ* 黄老哲理: This body of thinking dates to the late Warring states period (*Zhànguó* 戰國) of Chinese history (roughly 5th cent.-221 BCE) and the Han Dynasty 漢 (206 BCE-220 CE) periods. It is named after the two most important deities venerated, the "Yellow Emperor" *Huángdì* and *Lǎozi.*

37 Yáo 尧 and Shùn 舜 were two of the three mythic sage-rulers of antiquity during China's so-called Golden Age. They are mentioned in the *Shūjīng* 《書經》 (*Classic of History*) and were exalted by Confucius for their exemplary and sagely rule. According to Chinese tradition, Emperor Yáo is said to have ruled from approximately 2356-2256 BCE and to have relinquished the empire to his wise counselor Shùn, who ruled from roughly 2294-2184 BCE. In the *Zhōngyōng* 《中庸》 (*Doctrine of the Mean*), Yáo and Shùn are explicitly revered. As noted by Roger Ames and David Hall in *Focusing the Familiar: A Translation and Philosophical Interpretation of the Zhōngyōng* (2001), "*Confucius revered Yáo and Shùn as his ancestors and carried on their ways.*" A related passage referring to *Huáng Dì* 黄帝, *Yáo* 尧, and *Shùn* 舜 appears in the "Ten Wings," specifically the *Xì Cí Xià* 《系辞下》 section of the *Yìjīng. This text states that Huáng Dì, Yáo, and Shùn "simply wore their robes (yīshang* 衣裳*) as models for the people, and good order was thereby secured in the world,"* emphasizing moral example of humility and ritual propriety as the foundation of social harmony.

"*After the death of Shén Nóng* 神农*, there arose Huáng Dì* 黄帝*, Yáo* 尧*, and Shùn* 舜*. They carried through the (necessarily occurring) changes, so that the people did (what was required of them) without being wearied; yea, they exerted such a spirit-like transformation, that the people felt constrained to approve their (ordinances) as right. When a series of changes has run all its course, another change ensues. When it obtains free course, it will continue long. Hence it was that 'these (sovereigns) were helped by Heaven; they had good fortune, and their every movement was advantageous.' Huáng Dì* 黄帝*, Yáo* 尧*, and Shùn* 舜*, (simply) wore their upper and lower garments (as patterns to the people), and good order was secured all under heaven. The idea of all this was taken, probably, from Qián* 乾 *(☰/䷀) and Kūn* 坤 *(☷/䷁) (the first and eighth trigrams, or the first and second hexagrams)*" Adapted from Legge, (1882). *The Sacred Books of the East, vol. 16,* pp. 383-384.

[38] Saint from Heaven (*tiān tú shèng* 天徒聖).

[39] Saint-Master (*fū zǐ qí shèng* 夫子其聖)

[40] *Zhōngyōng* 《中庸》 (*Doctrine of the Mean)* refers to one of the Four Books of Confucian principles. Its origins may have been formulated in the *Classic of Rites (Lǐjì* 禮記). *Zhōngyōng* is also a general term in Confucianism, denoting moderation, balance, and appropriateness in thought and conduct. See Appendix III: *Etymological Glossary of Sage Principle Terms*, for a more detailed analysis of *yōng* 庸, *yì* 義, *rén* 仁, and *kèqì* 克己.

[41] This is Professor Cheng's reference to Chapter 20 of the *Dàodé jīng*, from his book *Lao-Tzu: My Words Are Very Easy to Understand*, translated by Tam Gibbs, (1981), pp. 74-75.

[42] This may correspond to Professor Cheng's interpretation of *Analects* 11.20: *"If, because a man's discourse appears solid and sincere, we allow him to be a good man, is he really a superior man? Or is his gravity only in appearance?"* Legge, (1883). *The Chinese Classics*, p. 59. This may also be compared with *Analects* 12.20, in which Confucius says: *"Now, the man of distinction is solid and straightforward, and loves righteousness. He examines people's words, and looks at their countenances. He is anxious to humble himself to others. Such a man will be distinguished in the country; he will be distinguished in the family. As to the man of notoriety, he assumes the appearance of virtue but his actions are opposed to it, and he rests in this character without any doubts about himself. Such a man will be heard of in the country, he will be heard of in the family"* Legge, (1883). *The Chinese Classics*, p. 66-67; as well as *Analects* 14.5 *"The virtuous will be sure to speak correctly, but those who speeches good may not always be virtuous. Men of principle are sure to be bold, but those who are bold may not always be men of principle"* Legge, (1883). *The Chinese Classics*, p. 75.

[43] Analects 13.3 *"If names be not correct, language is not in accordance with the truth of things. If language be not in accordance with the truth of things, affairs cannot be carried on to success"* Legge, (1883). *The Chinese Classics*, p. 69.

Chapter 2: 175 Words of the Sages[44]

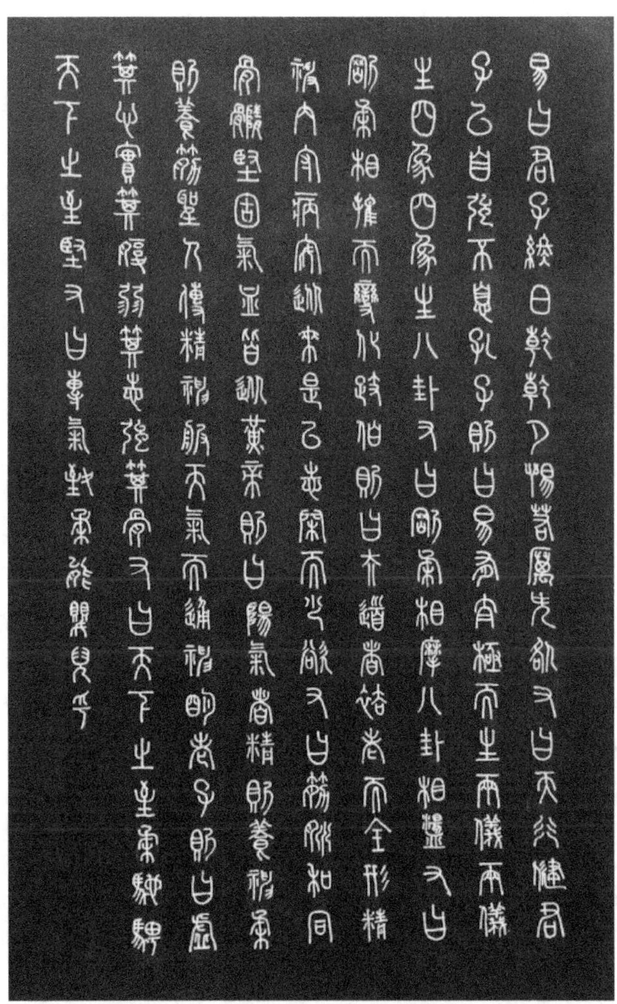

The 175 Sage Characters in Seal Script Form
created by Ed Young

The *Yìjīng* 《易经》(*Book of Changes*) states that "*the exemplary person rises up through the day and come evening, self-reflects so there is no harm.*" It also teaches that, "*The Heavens move with such vigor that the exemplary person is continuously energized.*"

The Confucian *Yì Zhuàn* 《易傳》(*Commentaries on The Book of Changes)* states that "*Tàijí gives birth to two modes, which in turn give birth to four images. The four images give birth to eight trigrams.*"[45] It further explains that "*when the hard and soft interact with each other, the eight trigrams swing with each other,*" and "*as the hard and soft respond to each other, they change and transform.*"

[In the Internal Medicine Classic *Huángdì Nèijīng Sùwèn* 《黄帝内經·素問》] Qíbó 岐伯 says: "*Now, those [who follow] the Way, they can drive away old age and they preserve their physical appearance* [...] *When essence and spirit are guarded internally, where could a disease come from? Hence, the mind is relaxed and one has few desires. The Heart is at peace and one has no fear.*" Qíbó also states "*The sinews and blood vessels are in harmony, [their] bones and marrow are solid and firm, and [their] qì* 氣 *and blood both follow [their usual course].*" In *The Internal Medicine Classic*, Emperor Huáng Dì 黄帝 says"*as for the yáng qì, if it is firm, it nourishes the spirit (shén* 神*;) if it is soft, it nourishes the sinews.* [...] *When the sages concentrated essence and spirit (jīng-shén), and when they ingested the qì of heaven, they communicated with the spirit brilliance (shénmíng* 神明*).*"

In the *Dàodé jīng* 《道德經》, Lǎozi teaches "*the Sage governs himself by relaxing the mind, reinforcing the abdomen, gentling the will, strengthening the bones,*"[46] Lǎozi also says: "*The softest in the world overcomes the strongest,*" and asks "*In concentrating the qì to attain softness, can one be like a baby?*"

Professor Cheng's Interpretations

易曰君子終日乾之夕惕着若无咎

The Book of Changes says: "The exemplary person[47] rises up through the day and come evening, self-reflects so there is no harm."

Interpretation:

The Book of "Changes" (*yì* 易)[48] is the name of the book created by the legendary ancient sage *Fúxī* 伏羲.[49] He lived before the dawn of recorded history, but the book was completed in the Zhou dynasty (*Zhōu dài* 周代 1046-256 BCE). It includes the principles of *Lǐ* 理, *Qì* 氣, and *Xiàng* 象; which contain the ideas of the constant (unchanging,) the exchanging and the changing.[50] The exemplary person is one whose virtues and talents are advanced because he spends the whole day advancing unceasingly yet at night self-reflects[51] on what he accomplished and considers whether he will be able to continue in the same way tomorrow. No harm can come from this attitude.

又曰天行健君子 自强不息

[The Book of Changes] also says: "The Heavens move with such vigor that the exemplary person is continuously energized."

Interpretation:

Proof of the vigor and constancy of Heaven is evidenced in its perpetual circadian (day-night) motion. Therefore, the exemplary person seeks to follow its example.

孔子則曰易有太極而生兩儀, 兩儀生四象四象生八卦

[*The Commentaries on the Book of Changes* by] Confucius says: "*In the Book of Changes the tàijí 太极 gives birth to two modes,*[52] *which in turn give birth to four images.*[53] *The four images give birth to eight trigrams.*"

Interpretation:

Confucius was the most outstanding scholar in Chinese history. As previously stated, the scholars that came after his time regarded him as "the Saintly Venerable Master." As for the text above, Confucius said "the *Book of Changes* speaks of *tàijí;*" *Tàijí* embodies the principle of *lǐ* 理, *qì* 氣, *xiàng* 象 as a process of differentiation.[54]

又曰剛柔相摩八卦相盪

[*The Commentaries on the Book of Changes* by] Confucius also says: "*When the hard and soft interact with each other, the eight trigrams swing with each other.*"

Interpretation:

"Hard and soft" indicates the nature and energy of *yáng* and *yīn* respectively. When *yáng* and *yīn* interact, the eight directions, synonymous with the Eight Trigrams, all begin to emerge.

又曰剛柔相推而變化

[The *Commentaries on the Book of Change* by] Confucius also says: "*As the hard and soft respond to each other, they change and transform.*"

Interpretation:

As the interaction between hard and soft continues, change takes place. This, then is the process of Change: from constant (no-change,) to exchange, and then change (*lǐ* 理, *qì* 氣, *xiàng* 象).

岐伯曰則夫道者能却老而全形

精神内守病安 從来是以志閑而少欲

[In the Internal Medicine Classic] Qíbó says: "*Now, those [who follow] the Way, they can drive away old age and they preserve their physical appearance.*"[55]

"When essence and spirit are guarded internally, where could a disease come from? Hence, the mind is relaxed and one has few desires. The Heart is at peace and one is not in fear."[56]

Interpretation:

Qíbó 岐伯 taught medical theory to Emperor Huángdì 黄帝.[57] His teachings became the medical classic *Sùwèn* 《素問》 called "Questions and Answers About Internal Medicine."[58] When Qíbó speaks of the Way, he means the principles of slowing the tendency toward senility and of preserving the youthfulness of one's form. What he means by "guarding the essence-spirit"[59] is that one should conserve one's energy inwardly rather than scattering it wastefully. If one is healthy there are no openings for sickness to penetrate.

岐伯曰 筋脉和同，骨髓坚固，氣血皆从

[In the *Internal Medicine Classic*] Qíbó says: " [...*their*] *sinews and vessels were in harmony, [their] bones and marrow were solid and firm, and* [*their*] *qì and blood both follow* [*their usual course*]."[60]

Interpretation:

When the essences (*jīng*) are full and the marrow is replenished, the blood and *qì* already follow each other in flowing.[61] This is proof of rejuvenation. "When the sinews and blood vessels are in harmony," means that the sinews and tendons move with the *qì* and therefore belong to *yáng* energy. The blood vessels move the blood and therefore belong to the *yīn* energy. The sinews are like electric wires and the blood vessels are like water pipes. For *qì* and blood to be in harmony is exactly the same as *yīn-yáng* mutually benefitting each other.[62]

黃帝曰則陽氣者精則養神柔則養筋
[In the *Internal Medicine Classic*] Emperor Huángdì says: "*As for the yang qi, if it is firm, it nourishes the spirit; if it is soft, it nourishes the sinews.*"[63]

聖人傳精神服天氣而通神明
"When the sages concentrated essence and spirit, and when they ingested the qi of heaven, they communicated with the spirit brilliance."[64]

Interpretation:

Emperor Huángdì, the Yellow Emperor, was the first emperor of the Chinese people in recorded history. His last name was Xuānyuán shì.[65] "Ceaseless life force" is *yáng qì* and might also be translated as "ceaselessly regenerating "spirit" (*shén*)." The combination of blood and *qì* condenses into "essence" (*jīng*). When this "essence" (*jīng*) grows strong, it undergoes a further transformation, condensing into "spirit" (*shén*). The words passed down by the sages concerning essence and spirit (*jīngshén*) are: begin by ingesting the breath of Heaven, and end with "divine brilliance" (*shénmíng* 神明).[66]

老子則曰虛其心實其腹弱其志强其骨

[In *Daode jing*] Lǎozi 老子 says: "[the sage governs himself by] relaxing the mind, reinforcing the abdomen, gentling the will, strengthening the bones."[67]

Interpretation:

Lǎozi (Lao-tzu) was the official keeper of the Imperial Archives of the Zhou dynasty. He wrote a book entitled *Dàodé jīng* (*Tao Teh Ching*),[68] which consists of about five thousand words. "Relaxing the mind"[69] means putting your mind in the state of *wúwéi*[70] or "non-doing." If the mind is in the state of *wúwéi*, it will naturally sink down with the breath *qì* to guard the *dāntián* 丹田.[71] The *dāntián* corresponds to the "womb" of the spirit of the Heart-mind. To "reinforce the abdomen"[72] means to sink the *qì* to the *dāntián* and thereby make it possible to strengthen the bones.[73]

又曰天下之至柔馳騁天下之至堅

[In *Dàodé jīng*] Lǎozi also says: "*The softest in the world overcomes the strongest.*"[74]

Interpretation:

Under Heaven, there is nothing softer[75] than wind and water. But if it gathers its energy and persists, wind will wear away brass, and water will penetrate stone. When this energy is concentrated, it can shake a mountain or turn the ocean over. There is no substance, no matter how hard, that can prevent this energy from penetrating.

又曰專氣致柔能嬰兒乎
[In *Dàodé jīng*] *Lǎozi* also says: "In concentrating the *qì* to attain softness, can one be like a baby?"[76]

Interpretation:
When *qì* is concentrated in the *dāntián* it travels through the system of membranes, reaching into the network of tendons and blood vessels, bringing them into harmony with each other. This is what is meant by concentrating the *qì* to bring about the softness (flexibility) of a child.

Ch. 2 Notes

[44] See Appendix III: *Etymological Glossary of Sage Principle Terms*, for a more detailed analysis of these characters.

[45] *Da Zhuan* 《大傳》 *(The Great Commentary)*

[46] Cheng & Gibbs, (1981). *Lao-Tzu: My Words Are Very Easy to Understand*, Chapter 3, p. 28-29.

[47] *"The exemplary person (jūnzǐ 君子) refers to one who is noble, mature, and cultivated. It is a central Confucian term denoting a morally refined and well-educated person who embodies ethical excellence in conduct and character. Jūnzǐ is variously translated as "gentleman," "ideal person," or "superior person."* Roger Ames renders *jūnzǐ* as "the exemplary person." Ames & Hall, (2001). *Focusing the Familiar a Translation and Philosophical Interpretation of the Zhongyong* and Appendix III: *Etymological Glossary of Sage Principle Terms*.

[48] *"As important as the Daoist and Confucian canons have been in articulating Chinese intellectual history, and as much as they may be appealed to as textual evidence for claims about early Chinese cosmology, perhaps no single text can compete with the Yìjīng 《易經》 (Book of Changes) in terms of the sustained interest it has garnered from successive generations of China's literati, or the influence it has exerted on Chinese self-understanding. The coordination of the relationship between the changing world and human experience constitutes the central axis of the Yìjīng."* See Ames, (2015). *The Great Commentary (Dazhuan 大傳) and Chinese Natural Cosmology*, pp. 1-2.

[49] Fú Xī 伏羲 (Fu Hsi) a legendary Chinese cultural hero and sovereign, traditionally dated to 2852-2738 BCE. He is credited with the invention of fishing and trapping, as well as with the creation of writing and the eight trigrams (*bāguà* 八卦), which later became foundational to the *Yìjīng* 《易經》 (*Book of Changes*).

[50] *Lǐ* 理–*Qì* 氣–*Xiàng* 象, will be discussed in Chapter 3. Briefly they represent a developmental movement from an unchanging, unifying "principle" (*lǐ* 理), associated with the primal unity of *wújí* 無極 ("non-differentiation"). Through differentiation, *tàijí* 太極 emerges, giving rise to *qì* 氣; the vital energy or "breath of life," generated through the dynamic interactions of *yīn-yáng*, heaven and earth. This process manifests in the phenomenal world as the diversity of changing forms and images (*xiàng* 象). See professor Cheng's explanation in Chapter 3 for further elaboration.

[51] "Self-reflects" The word *tì* 惕 is variously translated as "alert," "respectful," "cautious," "careful," "prudent," or "watchful," and can also convey fear or anxious attentiveness. The character shows the image of Heart–mind (*xīn* 心) with change (*yì* 易), suggesting a Heart capable of alert responsiveness to changing circumstances, like a flickering candle responding to the wind. Such cultivated self-awareness and attentiveness to change are essential qualities in the moral, self-reflection and spiritual cultivation of the mature person (*jūnzǐ* 君子).

---

52 Two modes (*liǎng yí* 兩儀) also translated as "two principles," or "two forms," and commonly refers to the fundamental duality of *yīn* 陰 and *yáng* 陽, or Heaven and Earth. These two principles are traditionally represented by the broken line (- -) for *yīn* and the unbroken line (—) for *yáng*, which exist in a dynamic, interconnected, and interdependent relationship. Each contains the seed of the other, and together they form the foundational basis of the sixty-four hexagrams of the *Yìjīng* 《易經》 (*Book of Changes*).

53 Four Images (*sì xiàng* 四象) relates to the four cardinal directions (see Chapter 3). Traditionally, the Four Symbolic Images are said to correspond to the four divisions of the 28 lunar mansions in Chinese astrology: the "Green Dragon" (*Qīng Lóng* 青龍) in the East represents Wood; the White Tiger (*Bái Hǔ* 白虎) in the West represents Metal; the Vermilion Bird (*Zhū Què* 朱雀) in the South represents Fire; and the Black Tortoise (*Xuán Wǔ* 玄武) in the North represents Water. These Four Images integrate cosmology, astrology, and the natural ecological forces of the world, reflecting classical Chinese orientation of the heavens, the cardinal directions, the seasons and the elemental phases.

54 See Chapter 3 entitled "Lǐ, Qì, Xiàng 理氣象."

55 Unschuld & Tessenow, (2011), p. 41.

56 ibid, p. 34.

57 Emperor Huang (*Huángdì* 黃帝), the "Yellow Emperor," is a legendary sage-king traditionally said to have lived during China's prehistoric era.

58 The *Huángdì Nèijīng* 《黃帝內經》 (*Yellow Emperor's Classic of Internal Medicine*) is considered the first major foundational Chinese medical classic. It integrates *yīn–yáng* theory, the Five Phases (*wǔxíng* 五行), and principles of diagnosis and treatment. Dating to the Han dynasty (206 BCE-220 CE), the text is structured as a series of questions and answers between the legendary Yellow Emperor (*Huángdì* 黃帝) and his physician, Qíbó.

59 Essence–Spirit (*jīng–shén* 精神) is composed of two characters: *jīng* 精, meaning essence, extract, vitality, seed or sperm; and *shén* 神, meaning spirit, mysterious, lively, expression, awesome, amazing, divine. Traditionally, *jīng* is considered more *yīn* in energy, relative to *shén* which possesses more *yáng* energy. Together, *jīng–shén* represents the central *yīn–yáng* relationship of life, embodying the unity of mind and body and expressing both physical vigor and spiritual consciousness. See Appendix III: *Etymological Glossary of Sage Principle Terms*, for a more detailed analysis of these characters.

60 Chapter 3 is entitled "*Discourse on How the Generative (Shēng) Qì Communicates with Heaven*" See Unschuld & Tessenow, (2011), p. 75.

---

61 Sinews and vessels (*jīn mài* 筋脈) refer to the flow of blood through the muscles and tendons. Alternatively, the muscles and tendons can be thought of as channels in themselves, through which vital energy circulates. Bone marrow (*gǔ suǐ* 骨髓) in East Asian medicine is said to be produced by the prenatal essences (*jīng* 精) stored in the Kidneys. Traditionally, the Kidney (adrenal/genitourinary system) is believed to store prenatal *jīng*, which generates the marrow that nourishes the bones. Marrow and bone exemplify the *yīn-yáng* relationship of soft and hard. The marrow is considered one of the extraordinary organs (*qíhéngfǔ* 奇恆腑), which also includes the spinal cord and brain. If Kidney essence is weak, the marrow and brain may be insufficient, preventing the spirit (*shén* 神) from shining fully.

62 East Asian medicine proposes a series of microcosms that reflect Nature as a whole. Using the Sage Principles, Professor Cheng is presenting the principle of mutual interdependence of *yīn-yáng*, expressed in the microcosmic forms of *jīng* 精 and *shén* 神, blood and *qì*, blood vessels and tendons, marrow and bone.

63 Unschuld renders *jīng* 精 here as "firm," in concordance with the *Nèijīng* interpretation by *Tàijí* grandmaster Gāo Jìwǔ 高纪武 (b.1942), who interprets *jīng* 精 as "strong" (*jiàng* 強) instead of "essence." This interpretation in this context aligns with Professor Cheng's reading of *jīng* as a fundamental *yīn* element both firm *and* soft within the transformational process: the essence (*jīng* 精) is the firm root or seed that generates *yáng qì* 陽氣 which, with cultivation, nourishes mental clarity and flourishes as spiritual power. This interpretation is consistent with the overarching theme of the *Nèijīng* Chapter 3, "*Discourse on How the Generative Qì Communicates with Heaven,*" which emphasizes how the sage harmonizes with seasonal and circadian cycles to nourish *yáng qì*, promote health, and ward off illness. See Unschuld & Tessenow, (2011), p. 70.

64 ibid. p. 61.

65 Xuānyuán Shì 軒轅氏 (Hsien Yuen Shih).

66 Divine Brilliance (*shénmíng* 神明), translated also as "spiritual clarity," represents the creative energy that emanates from the spirit (*shén* 神). For more on the practice of "swallowing the *qì* of Heaven," see Appendix I: *Parting Words of Professor Cheng* and Footnote 304.

67 Lǎozi 老子, Chapter 3, in *Lao-Tzu: My Words Are Very Easy to Understand. Lectures on the Tao Teh Ching:* Cheng & Gibbs, (1981), pp. 28-29.

68 *Dàodé jīng* 《道德經》 the Lǎozi classic of the Way and Power/Virtue.

69 "Relaxing the Mind" (*xū qí xīn* 虛其心) In Chinese, *xū* 虛 means empty or unoccupied, implying "relaxed," or uncluttered, while *xīn* 心 represents both Heart and mind. *Xū qí xīn* 虛其心 therefore refers to a mind that is calm, open, and not preoccupied. See further discussion in Chapter 5.

70 *Wúwéi* 無為 literally "non-action" or "without doing" is an important concept in Daoism, presented in the *Lǎozi (Dàodéjīng). Wúwéi* refers to natural, spontaneous, and "selfless" action or action that is free from bias, manipulation, coercion, and unnecessary struggle.

Daniel Schrier, editor's note: *Wúwéi* is not inactivity, but "effortless," "non-interfering" action, doing nothing extra and only what is necessary. It is an existential principle and contemplative practice expressed through apophatic, quietistic meditation: "contentless," "non-conceptual," and "non-dual." It involves de-conditioning, detachment, and disengagement, ceasing what obstructs one's "innate nature" (*xìng* 性) and restoring one's original alignment to and with the Dao. Often misunderstood as "passivity" or "indulging desire," *wúwéi* is linked with "desirelessness" (*wúyù* 無欲), "non-contention" (*wúzhēng* 無爭), "non-knowing" (*wúzhī* 無知), and "suchness" (*zìrán* 自然). In practice, *wúwéi* culminates in *zìrán* which is sometimes rendered in English as Daoist Quietism.

71 *Dāntián* 丹田 (tan-t'ien) An important concept in *Tàijí* practice, the term literally means "cinnabar field." (See Chapter 9 and Appendix III: *Etymological Glossary of Sage Principle Terms*, for a more detailed analysis of these characters.)

72 "Reinforce the Abdomen" (*shí qí fù* 實其腹). *Shí* 實 can be translated as "solid," "full," "to fill," or "fruit." In this context in the *Lǎozi (Dàodé jīng)*, it contrasts with *xū* 虛 ("empty"), signifying the act of filling, reinforcing, ripening or solidifying the abdomen/belly.

73 "Gentling the Will" (*ruò qí zhì* 弱其志). The character *ruò* 弱 is illustrated by the image of two tender baby birds' wings, conveys softness or weakness. *Zhì* 志, translated as "will," "drive," "ambition," "aspiration," or "desire," depicts a seedling rising from the ground, symbolizing insistence or determination in one's thoughts and actions. In *Tàijí* practice, *zhì* may be understood as carrying more force than *yì* 意 ("intention" or "focused attention") and therefore something to avoid.

74 Chapter 43, in *Lao-Tzu: My Words Are Very Easy to Understand. Lectures on the Tao Teh Ching:* Cheng & Gibbs (1981), p. 149.

75 *Róu* 柔 is often translated as "soft," "flexible," "pliant," "supple," "yielding." See Appendix III: *Etymological Glossary of Sage Principle Terms*, for a more detailed analysis of these characters.

76 Chapter 10, in Cheng & Gibbs, (1981), *Lao-Tzu: My Words Are Very Easy to Understand: Lectures on the Tao Teh Ching*, pp. 46-47.

Note: "resiliency" has been replaced with "softness" to align with the term 柔 used in previous quotes. Professor Cheng's commentary on Chapter 10 (p. 46) explains that "concentrating the *qì*" refers to breathing. Regarding "attaining softness," Qíbó 岐伯 advised, "let the circulatory system of blood and *qì* flow freely." This reflects Lǎozi's emphasis on the cultivation of *qì*, as further illustrated in Chapter 55: "*the sinews are soft yet the grip is firm*" and "*reverse old age and become like a child.*"

Chapter 3: Lǐ, Qì, Xiàng 理氣象 & the Eight Trigram Bāguà 八卦 Sequence

In the commentaries on *the Book of Changes*, Confucius states:

河出图洛出书圣人则之
"The Hé-River gave forth the map, and the Luò (Lo), the writing, (both of) which the sages took advantage."[77]

With these words, the sages pointed to the fact that the *bāguà* 八卦 (eight trigrams) of Fúxī 伏羲,[78] upon which the *Yìjīng* 《易經》 *(Book of Changes)*[79] was based, in turn had its beginning in the Hétú River Diagram (Figure 2)[80] and the Luò Writing (Figure 3).[81]

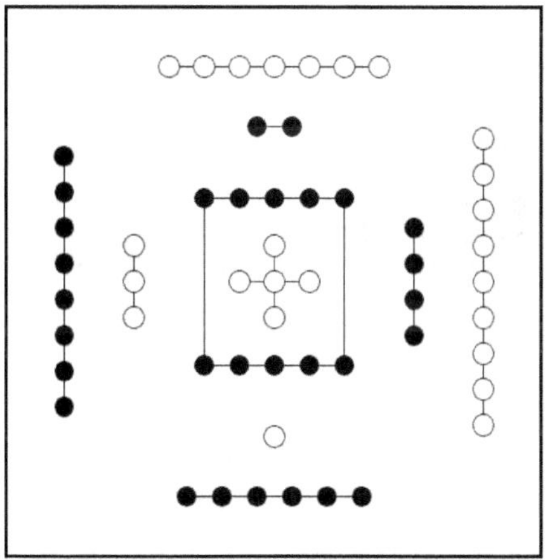

Figure 2: The Hétú River Diagram

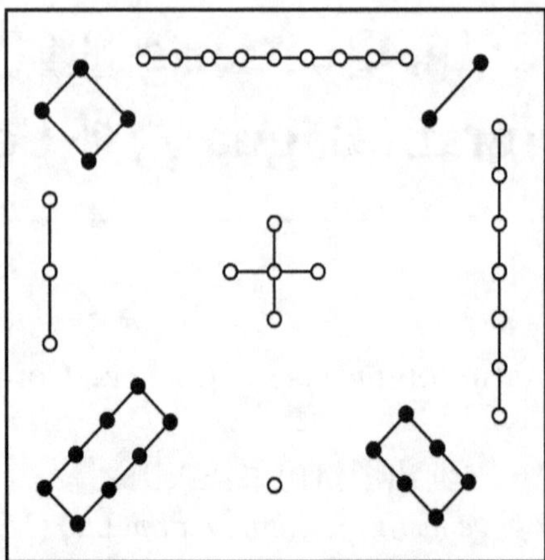

Figure 3: The Luòshū Book of Luò

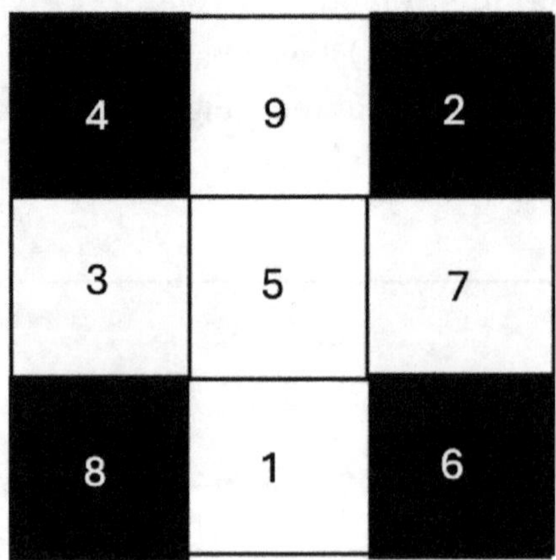

Figure 4: Magic Square

These symbolic arrangements are ancient, their origin veiled in myth. The diagrams are comprised of *yáng;* white (empty) circles and *yīn;* Black (solid) circles with connecting lines. Each component has its own name and symbolic attributes.

Lǐ 理 Qì 氣 Xiàng 象

The origin of the *Tàijí* diagram (seen in Figure 1) is based on the three principles of *Lǐ* 理, *Qì* 氣, *Xiàng* 象.

Lǐ 理[82] represents the unifying principle of constant interactivity between *yīn-yáng*.[83] The descent of *yángqì* 陽氣 of Heaven and the ascent of *yīnqì* 陰氣 of Earth and their harmonious union results in the creation of everything. *Lǐ* is the constant relativity of Heaven and Earth preserved in the outer shell of the *Tàijí* diagram and the hidden connection between the dots.

Qì 氣[84] is represented by the white circles in the River Diagram and correspond to *yáng* odd numbers.[85] Qì corresponds to Spirit (*shén* 神),[86] Sky/Heaven (*tiān* 天) and *yáng*.[87] Generally, there are three kinds of *qì*:

- *Tiānqì* 天氣[88] or *qì* of the atmospheric weather (heavenly *qì*)
- *Xuèqì* 血氣[89] or *qì* of the blood (circulation)
- *Jīngqì* 精氣[90] or congenital *qì* also known as *yuánqì* (original source *qì*).

In the Heavens, *tiānqì*, represents the air that all living things breathe. In human beings, it is represented by the *xuèqì* or *qì* of blood circulation. Its function is to nourish and maintain the body's warmth.[91] In Earth, this *qì* is called *jīngqì* or congenital *qì* which in Chinese physiology is also called the primal *qì* (*yuánqì*)[92] and is recognized as the original source material of life in humans. The origin of a human life comes from the union of father's and mother's *jīng*-essence, representing Heaven and Earth respectively. During the time of intercourse, the *jīngqì* (male/*yáng* semen) is brought forth and combines with the female/*yīn jīngqì* (ovum.) According to

Chinese Sage Principles, humans emerge from this *yīn-yáng* relationship represented by the term *jīngshén* 精神,[93] which will be explained separately.

Xiàng 象[94], represented by the black circles in the River and Luo diagrams, corresponds to the even *yīn* numbers,[95] Earth, material substance and everything in the universe that has form and shape. Anything that has form is called *xiàng* and is associated with Earth *yīn*.

Now it can be seen that the essence of the River Diagram and Book of Luo refers to the principles of *Lǐ Qì Xiàng* 理氣象 (seen in Figure 5). These same three, though represented by different symbols, are exactly the same components that form the *tàijí* diagram

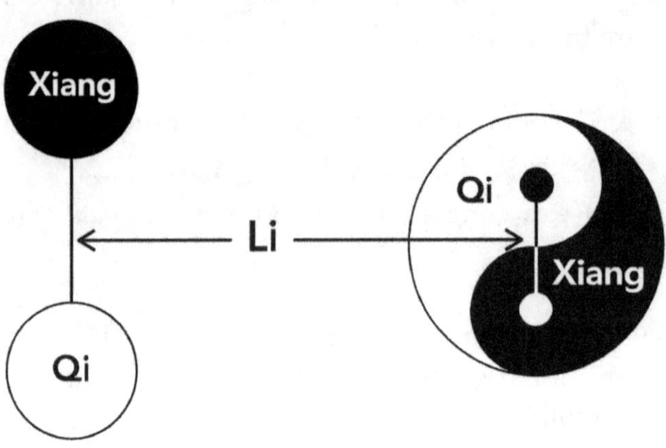

***Figure 5: Lǐ Qì Xiàng* 理氣象**
Based on Sketches by Cheng Man-Ch'ing

Here's a simplified summary:

- *Lǐ* 理 is "oneness" (unity principle). The continuity and endless flow of change (*biàntōng*)[96] generated by this oneness is called *Wújí* which means "without limits."[97]
- *Wújí* includes the great atmosphere (heavenly *qì*). It is called *Hùndùn*[98] which means primal chaos as shown in the diagram by the outer line encircling the *yīn-yáng*.
- *Hùndùn* exists before the separation of the clear and muddy (light and heavy). When separation and differentiation take place, the result is *tàijí*[99] (great ultimate or extreme polarity).

According to the *Yìjīng*, once the clear (insubstantial, Heavenly) and muddy (substantial, Earthly) of *tàijí* are distinguished, it is called "oneness gives birth to two"[100] as shown in Figure 6 below.

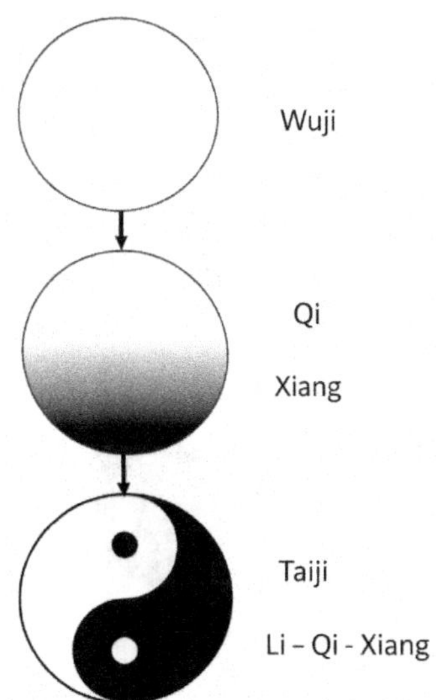

Figure 6: Wújí produces Tàijí

The Paired Modes *Liǎngyí* 兩儀

易有太极，是生两仪，两仪生四象，四象生八卦

"In [the book of] Changes, there is the Supreme Polarity, (tàijí 太極), which generates the Two Modes (liǎngyí 兩儀). The Two Modes generate the Four Images, (sìxiàng 四象) and the Four Images generate the Eight Trigrams (bāguà 八卦)."[101]

This differentiation (of *yīn-yáng*) is called the "Paired Modes" (*liǎngyí*).[102] Now the empty, white represents *qì*, *yáng* and Heaven. The black represents *xiàng*, *yīn* and Earth. The connecting line that maintains their constant interaction is *lǐ*. It is this principle of inter-relationship, which connects the *qì* and *xiàng*, that represents the "marriage" of Heaven and Earth. *Lǐ* governs the beginning of Heaven and Earth's interactions. Sometimes (aspects of) Heaven and Earth may be destroyed and yet (by definition) the presence of the constant whole will still persist.

The term "Paired Modes" (sometimes translated as "Two Forms") is used when describing the abstract relationship between Heavenly and Earthly functions, as in the two fundamental trigrams of Heaven (three solid lines) and Earth (three broken lines).[103]

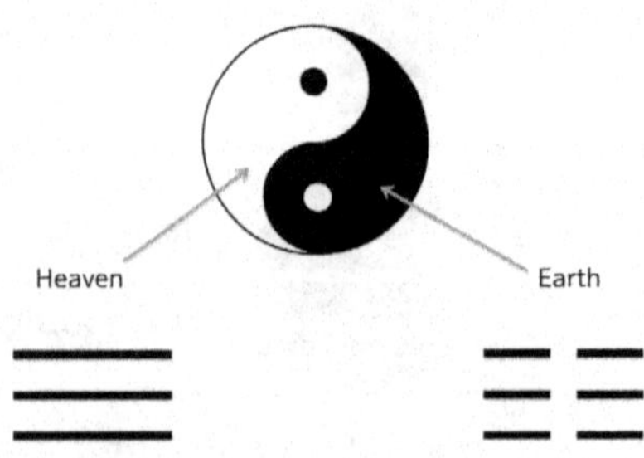

Figure 7: Heaven and Earth (the two modes)

In referring to Heavenly *Yáng* as the male aspect, and Earthly *Yīn* as the female aspect, this couple is said to have intercourse, producing offspring (seen in Figure 7).[104] When this pair interact (as husband and wife), they produce the first two offspring, called Water and Fire.[105] When the *yáng* or male influence is predominant (it provides the solid *yáng* line within the broken lines), the product will be Water. Conversely, when the *yīn* or female influence is predominant (it provides the *yīn* broken line within the yang solid lines), the product will be Fire. This is why the classics say Heaven gives birth to Water, and Earth gives birth to Fire (seen in Figure 8).

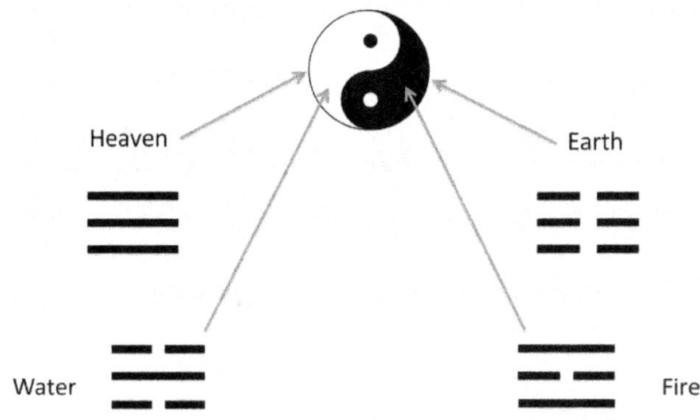

Figure 8: The Four Symbolic Images (Sìxiàng 四象)[106]

The transformation of the paired modes into the Four Symbols is the first stage of evolution in the trigram series. The Four Symbols are illustrated as follows (see Figure 9).

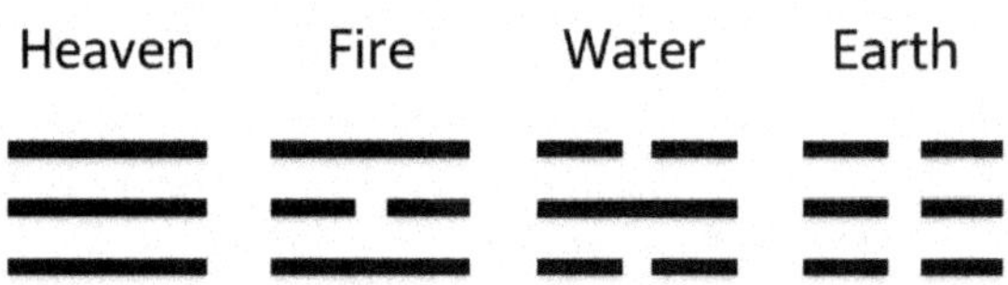

Figure 9: The Four Symbols

To consider the meaning of the Four Symbols leads to the study known as "Learning from the Symbols" (*fǎ xiàng* 法象)[107] In its most abstract sense, this learning (*fǎ* 法) may be interpreted as reflecting Lǎozi's words:

"Man learns from Earth
Earth learns from Heaven
Heaven learns from Dao
Dao learns from Nature"[108]

Most people are familiar with the phrase; "a picture is worth a thousand words." This refers to one's ability to study a picture and learn from it. To "learn from the forms" requires a similar exercise of observation and consideration. Following the laws (*fǎ* 法) of Nature, this study concerns three categories (Heaven, Earth, Dao). Of the primary forms, the greatest model of all is Heaven and Earth, which is always visible.

The Four Directions and the Four Corners

The Four Symbols are arranged as four directions and correspond to the movement of the four seasons (see Figure 10).[109]

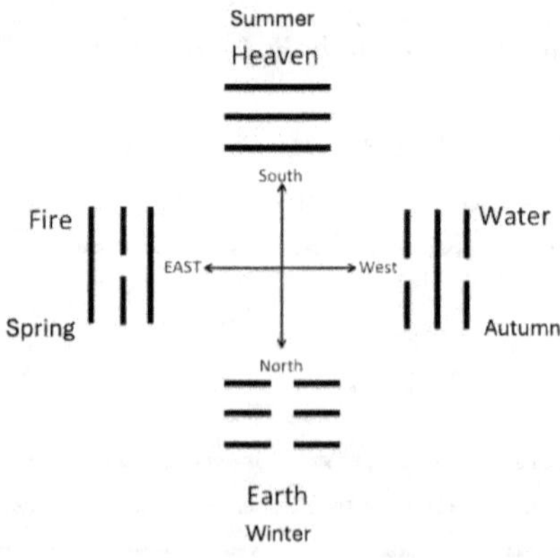

Figure 10: Four Directions

Heaven and Earth give birth again to two additional generations of symbols making a total of Eight Symbolic Images (the eight trigrams *bāguà* 八卦). As discussed above, the first four primary symbols correspond to the four directions and four seasons while the next two pairs of symbols correspond to the "four corners" and four additional directions (see Figure 11).[110] These last four symbolic images, which make up the "four corners," are called Mountain, Stream, Thunder and Wind.[111]

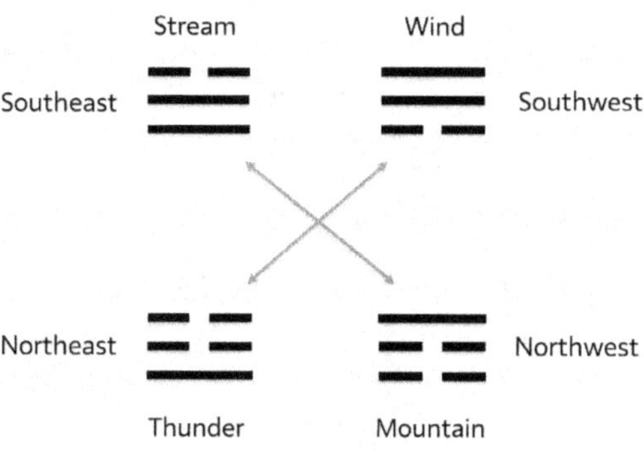

Figure 11: Four Corners

This is the end of the series generated by Heaven and Earth's interactions, and the total is called the Eight Symbols *(bāxiàng* 八象), although it is commonly referred to as the Eight Trigrams (*bāguà* 八卦).[112] Each of the Eight Symbols is unique and alive in itself and can interact with the others producing the 64 Hexagrams of the *Yìjīng* (see Figure 12).[113]

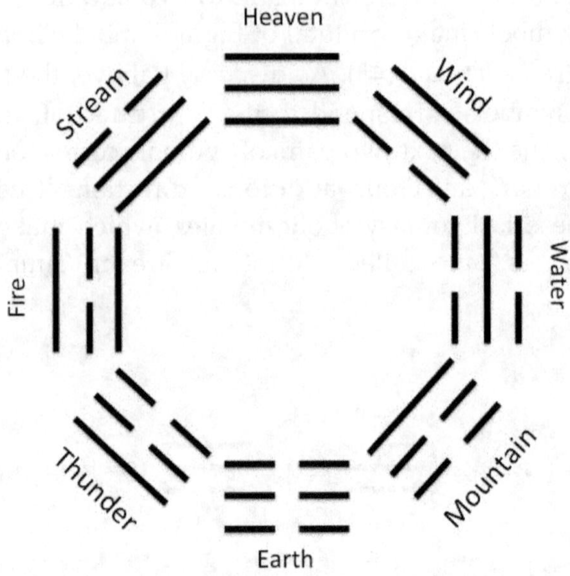

Figure 12: Eight Trigrams (Bāguà 八卦)

Just as there is a communication between Heaven and Earth, Mountain and Stream also interact. In the case of the latter, communication can be interpreted as meaning that no matter how massive the mountain is, water always penetrates. For instance, just as water's action penetrates the mountain in the form of a spring, its *qì* finds a path down the mountain. This is what makes it a "living mountain." But if water meets solid rock and cannot penetrate it, the rock is "dead," and a mountain of such solid impenetrable rock is considered a "dead mountain." Also, water which is stagnant and unmoving is considered "dead water." It has no *qì*, or motive force. This kind of water will not even penetrate a living mountain. But if the water is lively and if the mountain is living, then the water will penetrate and flow and there will be an interchange of *qì* between water and mountain (see Figure 13).

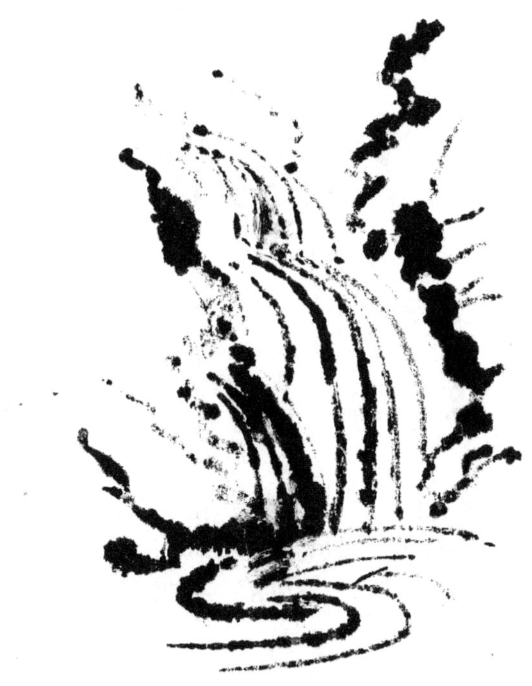

Figure 13: Living Mountain/ Living Water
Illustration by Ed Young

The final two symbolic images generated by the interaction of Heaven and Earth are called Wind and Thunder which also communicate with each other. And just as Fire and Water are opposites, so too Wind and Thunder will cause turbulence and conflict when they move against each other. The relationship of Wind and Thunder is that of mutual invasion, each pressuring and trying to overcome the other[114] (see Figure 14).

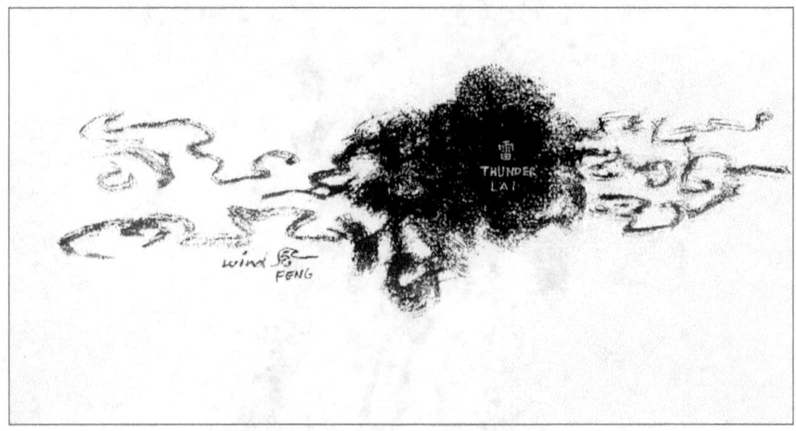

Figure 14: Thunder within Wind
Illustration by Ed Young

This is the end of the trigram series. The complete series is called the Eight Trigrams (*Bāguà*) which in turn generate the 64 hexagrams that make up the *Yìjīng* (see Figure 15 below).

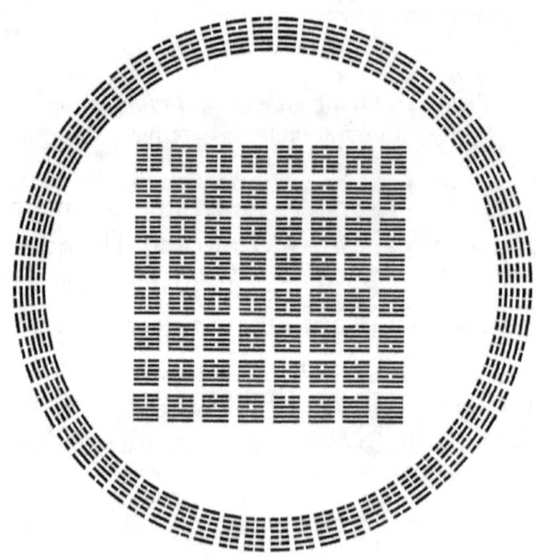

Figure 15: 64 Hexagrams of the Yìjīng

Additional Commentary on the Numerology of the Eight Trigrams *Bāguà* Generations

Traditionally the sages numbered the sequence of changes according to the order of birth, with odd numbers corresponding with *yáng* (father) and even numbers corresponding to *yīn* (mother) (see Figure 16).[115]

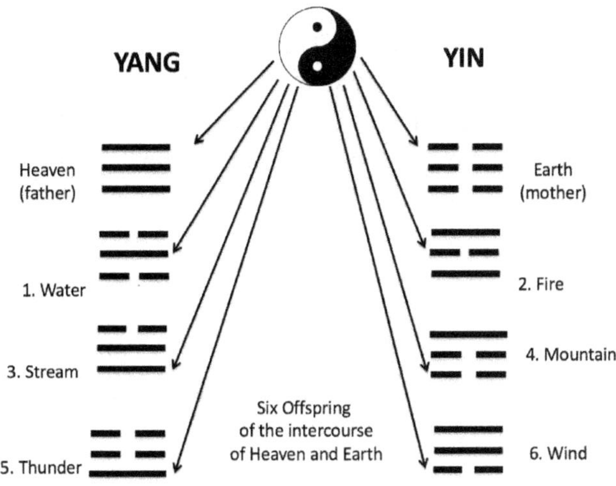

Figure 16: Numerology of the Trigrams.

The sequence of "birthing" of the offspring of Heaven (father) and Earth (mother) is as follows (odd numbers are *yáng*, even numbers are *yīn*):

1. Heaven (*Qián* 乾) corresponding to odd *yáng* numbers and merging with Earth (*Kūn* 坤) gives its middle *yáng* line to Earth to give birth to the first offspring which is Water (*Kǎn* 坎).
2. Earth (*Kūn* 坤), corresponding to even *yīn* numbers gives a *yīn* line to the middle of Heaven to produce the second offspring Fire (*Lí* 離).

3. The third offspring, being an odd *yáng* number, corresponds to Heaven this time giving its *yáng* line to the top of Earth to produce the third offspring called Mountain (*Gèn* 艮).
4. Heaven and Earth have intercourse again and produce the fourth offspring, an even number, which puts it in the realm of Earth. Earth gives a *yīn* line to the top of Heaven producing Stream (*Duì* 兌).
5. The fifth offspring (odd *yáng* number) means that Heaven is the dominant influence in intercourse, sharing a *yáng* line to the bottom of Earth generating Thunder (*Zhèn* 振).
6. The sixth and final offspring in the series (even *yīn* number 6) means it's under the influence of Earth sharing a *yīn* line to the bottom of Heaven giving birth to Wind (*Xùn* 巽).

Application of the *yīn-yáng* numerology (even/odd) then generates the Later Heavenly re-arrangement (*hòutiān* 後天) of the *bāguà* (see Figure 17).

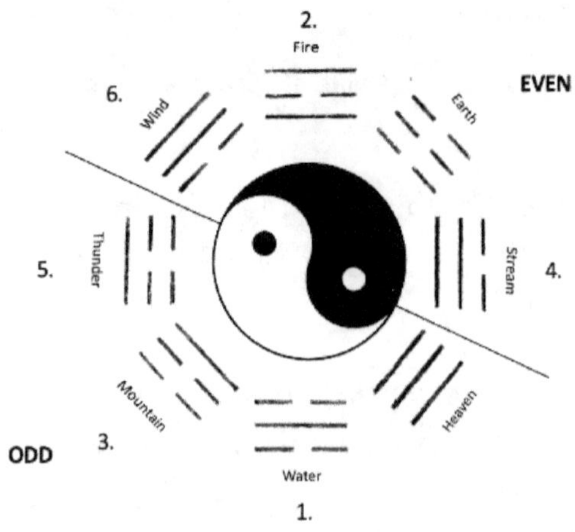

Figure 17: Later Heaven Hòutiān 後天 Bāguà[116]

The combination and interchange of these eight trigrams establishes the basis of the generation of the sixty-four hexagrams in the *Yìjīng* 《易經》 (*Book of Changes*).

Ch. 3 Notes

---

77 From *The Great Treatise* (*Yì Zhuàn* 易傳 or *Dà Zhuàn* 大傳, "Great Commentary") on the *Yìjīng*, traditionally attributed to Confucius (*Kǒngzǐ* 孔子). Adapted from Legge (1882), *The Sacred Books of the East, vol. 16*, p. 374.

[78] Fúxī (Fu Hsi) 伏羲 was considered the first mythical emperor of China. He is said to have discovered the eight Chinese trigrams (*bāguà* 八卦) used in divination, while meditating by the Yellow River. Scholars have long debated how the River Diagram and Luo Book inspired the trigrams; in this chapter, Professor Cheng offers his perspective on this connection. In addition to his role in divination, the legendary Fúxī is said to have been the father of Chinese writing and domesticated animals, and he taught his people to cook, fish with nets, and hunt using weapons made of iron, reflecting the neolithic origins of Chinese culture.

[79] The Eight Trigrams (*bāguà* 八卦), are considered the basic components of the *Yìjīng* 《易經》 sixty-four hexagrams. As Roger T. Ames observes, "*As important as the Daoist and Confucian canons have been in the articulation of Chinese intellectual history, and as much as they may be appealed to as textual evidence for claims about early Chinese cosmology perhaps no single text can compete with the Yìjīng* 《易經》 *(Book of Changes) in terms of the sustained interest it has garnered from succeeding generations of China's literati, and the influence it has had on Chinese self-understanding.*" See Ames (2015), *The Great Commentary (Dazhuan* 大傳*) and Chinese Natural Cosmology*.

[80] *Hétú* 河圖 literally "*River Diagram,*" also translated as "*River Map*" or "*River Chart.*"

[81] *Luòshū* 洛書 literally "*Luo Writing(s)*" or "*Book of Luò.*"

[82] *Lǐ* 理 – has many interrelated meanings depending on context in Chinese language: texture; patterns, grain (of wood or stone); intrinsic order; reason, principle, logic, science, truth. *Lǐ* ensures that *yīn-yáng* are always in relationship and always relative to each others.

[83] See appendix for Professor Cheng's original notes and diagram of *Lǐ Qì Xiàng* 理氣象 that extrapolate the graphic representation of the relationship of *Lǐ Qì Xiàng* in the *tàijí* 太極 symbol.

[84] Qì 氣 (ch'i) is often translated as "vital energy." The character depicts rice being cooked and releasing steam, symbolizing a dynamic, transformative force. See Appendix III: *Etymological Glossary of Sage Principle Terms*, for a more detailed analysis of these characters.

[85] Odd numbers correspond to *yáng* and even numbers correspond to *yīn* in Daoist numerology.

[86] *Shén* 神 associated with *expression, awareness, charisma,* and *spirit*. It is considered the more *yáng*, forming a complementary pair with *jīng* 精, the essence, which is considered more *yīn*. Together, *jīng-shén* 精神 is a term used to describe the body-mind unity in East Asian medicine and philosophy.

[87] *Yáng* 陽 ideogram showing the sunny hillside, refers to the atmospheric qualities associated with sunny, clear, but also masculine, explicit, visible (also positive electric charge).

---

88 *Tiānqì* 天氣 (*t'ien-ch'i*) "Heavenly Qì" refers to the effects of air quality, climate and weather on our health.

89 *Xuèqì* 血氣 (*hsueh* ch'i) ("blood *qì*") refers to the metabolic effects carried in blood circulation.

90 *Jīngqì* 精氣 ("essence *qì*") here refers to genital *qì* that provides vital life force given to us by our parents

91 According to East Asian medicine, the *shén* 神 (spirits) are carried in the *xuè* 血 (blood). Likewise, there is also an important *yin-yáng* relationship between blood and *qì* 氣: the blood is said to carry the *qì*, while the *qì* is said to move and circulate the blood, reflecting their interdependent and mutually nourishing functions.

92 *Yuánqì* 元氣: *"Source Qì"* or *"Original Qì"* is a fundamental concept in East Asian medicine. It is also generally translated as *vigor* or *strength*. In Chinese, the related term *jīngqì* 精氣 (essence-*qì*) can refer to semen or sperm, similar to how these terms are sometimes used interchangeably in English. *Yuánqì*, however, has a broader meaning, referring to a person's original or innate *qì*, regardless of gender. Thus, *yuánqì* can be interpreted as the eggs within the ovaries as well as the sperm, encompassing the fundamental reproductive potential and vital essence in both males and females.

93 *Jīngshén* 精神 as discussed in the previous chapter, is an important term in Chinese medicine and early Daoist texts. It refers to the body–mind–spirit unity present in all living, sentient beings.

94 *Xiàng* 象 (hsiang) translated as "shape;" "form;" "appearance;" "likeness" (such as a portrait); "image;" "snapshot;" "phenomenon;" or the outward expression of anything, including weather patterns and heavenly bodies.

The ideogram 象 depicts a large elephant (Oracle script:), conveying a sense of something substantial in contrast to the insubstantial qualities of air/steam/*qì* 氣. In *yīn-yáng* philosophy, the complementary and interdependent poles are often characterized as heavy and light, substantial and insubstantial, still and active. In *tàijí* 太極 practice, when we speak of empty and full, it is important to remember that these are relative terms reflecting an ongoing process so that it may be better to say "emptying in order to fill" and "filling in order to empty."

95 *Yīn* 陰 ideogram shows a cloudy hillside. It also relates to the atmospheric qualities associated with overcast weather; cloudy; shady; as well as the feminine; moon; implicit; hidden; genitalia.

[96] *Biàntōng* 變通: Flux and flow, change and continuity; free-flowing change; pragmatic; flexible; adapting one's actions to different situations or circumstances. This important concept appears frequently in the *Yìjīng* 《易經》 and is considered a fundamental aspect of Chinese thought. As the *Dà Zhuàn* 《大傳》 (Great Commentary on the *Yìjīng*) notes: *"The Master asked rhetorically, 'Does not the person who understands the course of flux and transformation in fact have insight into the workings of the spiritual?'"* See Ames (2015), *The Great Commentary (Dazhuan 大傳) and Chinese Natural Cosmology*.

[97] *Wújí* 無極 literally without limits is said to come before the division into *yīn-yáng* (*Tàijí* 太極 the ultimate limits of relativity.)

[98] *Hùndùn* 混沌 in Chinese mythology means primal chaos or formless mass before creation; it also means spontaneity or "innocent as a baby." (See *Zhuāngzǐ* Chapter 7 and Appendix III: *Etymological Glossary of Sage Principle Terms*, for a more detailed analysis of these characters.)

[99] *Tàijí* 太極: *Tài-* extreme, supreme *jí-* "limit" or "pole." The *tàijí* symbol is a graphic depiction of the interaction between *yīn-yáng*. The dots in the center of each indicating their mutually generating relationship.

[100] *Lǎozi* Chapter 42: "Dao gives birth to one, one gives birth to two, two gives birth to three, three gives birth to the ten thousand things."

[101] Adapted from Legge (1882), *The Sacred Books of the East, vol. XVI*, p. 12.

[102] *Liángyí* 兩儀 - Refers to the Heaven and Earth / *yáng* and *yīn* relationship. *Yí* is translated as "apparatus," "rites," "appearance," or "modes." *Liángyí* is also sometimes written as *liángxiàng* 兩象, meaning "two forms." Professor Cheng uses both terms. The word *liáng* ("two" in this context) should be distinguished from *èr* 二 (the number 2), which implies two separate entities. *Liáng* is better understood as "couple" or "paired," as in "drawn to each other."

[103] In some texts the "Two Modes" (*liángyí* 兩儀) are represented by a single solid line (— ; *yáng*) and a broken line (- -; *yīn*), which then generate the Four Symbols (*sìxiàng* 四象), represented by two lines. However, Professor Cheng explains the generation of the Eight Trigrams (*bāguà* 八卦) using a "family generations" method. See Appendix III: *Etymological Glossary of Sage Principle Terms*, for a more detailed analysis of these characters.

[104] The reader is cautioned not to take the words "male" and "female" too literally here. These relationships are being spoken of in the relative sense of *yáng* and *yīn* qualities of hard and soft, active and still that exist within all living things.

[105] We have chosen the use of the term "mode" to describe the primary two forms which Professor Cheng refers to later in this chapter as the "parents" as distinguished from the succeeding six generations.

---

106 *Sìxiàng* (*ssu-hsiang*) 四象, or four symbolic images ("Four emblematic symbols" as translated by James Legge) is sometimes confusingly called the "Four Forms." Traditionally the four images or symbols are said to correspond to the four divisions of the 28 constellations in Chinese astrology, namely: the Green Dragon (*qīnglóng* 青龍), White Tiger (*báihǔ* 白虎), Vermilion Bird (*zhūquè* 朱雀), and the Black Tortoise (*xuánwǔ* 玄武). These four symbols relate to the four primary directions respectively: East, West, South, and North.

107 *Fǎ xiàng* 法象, to learn from the forms or literally to follow (or live according to) the forms is mentioned in the Confucian commentary on the *Yìjīng* 《易經》 Chapter 1 法象莫大乎天地 变通莫大乎四时，县象著明莫大乎日月 "*Therefore of all things that furnish models and visible figures there are none greater than heaven and earth; of things that change and extend an influence (on others) there are none greater than the four seasons; of things suspended (in the sky) with their figures displayed clear and bright, there are none greater than the sun and moon*" see Legge (1882), *The Sacred Books of the East, vol. XVI*, p. 12.

108 This quote is from *Lǎozi* Chapter 25 人法地, 地法天, 天法道, 道法自然 (fǎ 法 implies: "to learn from," "to follow the ways of," "to model oneself after," "to be inspired by," "to be fashioned after"). Adapted from translation by Taoist Master Alfred Huang (1998), *The Complete I-Ching: The Definitive Translation,* p. 53.

109 In terms of sage principles, both the *Huángdì Nèijīng* and the Confucian commentaries on the *Yìjīng* refer to the Sage living in accord with the circadian cycles of Day/Night (*yīn-yáng*) and the four seasons. For example, *Sùwèn* 1 (7-3) "*They adapted themselves to [the regularity] of yīn-yáng and they lived in harmony with the four seasons*" Unschuld & Tessenow (2011), p. 43. Similarly, see the commentary on *Yìjīng* 《易經》, Chapter 1 (footnote 107).

110 In terms of trigrams, the picture can be described as follows (see Figures 10 & 11). Two trigrams are at the origin of all others, they represent the father and mother: *Qián* 乾, related to Heaven and composed of three solid *yáng* lines, symbolizing pure *yáng*; and *Kūn* 坤, related to Earth and composed of three broken *yīn* lines, symbolizing pure *yīn*. *Qián* and *Kūn* joined to give birth to the other trigrams, two of which are especially important for the alchemist: *Kǎn* 坎 and *Lí* 離. The inner line of *Kǎn* (a *yáng* line enclosed between two *yīn* lines) and the inner line of *Lí* (a *yīn* line enclosed within two *yáng* lines) are True *yáng* and True *yīn*, respectively. Their multiple meanings and functions cannot be fully described here. Suffice it to say that they represent the trace and union of the father and mother, and above all express a fundamental principle of interdependence: there is no *yīn* without *yáng*, and vice versa, or there would be sterility." Robinet (1997), *The World Upside Down: Essays on Taoist Internal Alchemy,* p. 4

---

[111] Mountain (*shān* 山), Stream/Marsh (*duì* 兌), Wind (*fēng* 風), Thunder (*léi* 雷). These characters are interpretations of the original eight trigrams listed in the *Yìjīng*: *Kǎn* 坎 (☵), *Kūn* 坤 (☷), *Lí* 離 (☲), *Qián* 乾 (☰), *Xùn* 巽 (☴), *Zhèn* 振 (☳), *Gèn* 艮 (☶), *Duì* 兌 (☱). See Appendix III: *Etymological Glossary of Sage Principle Terms*, for a more detailed analysis of these characters.

[112] The Eight Trigrams, or *Bāguà* 八卦 are the basic components of the ***Yìjīng's*** sixty-four hexagrams.

[113] This arrangement of the eight trigrams is known as the Early (former, or pre-heaven) Heaven arrangement (*xiāntiān* 先天) of the *Yìjīng*. It is said to have been organized by the legendary sage Fúxī and is arranged according to the ideal *yīn-yáng* relationships of the four pairs of trigrams; heaven and earth, fire and water, mountain and stream, wind and thunder.

[114] It is interesting to note that the two mutually influencing pairs (mountain-stream and thunder-wind are important hexagrams 31䷞ and 32䷟ located halfway in the 64 hexagram *bāguà* that separate the so-called "Upper Canon" from the "Lower Canon." Hexagram 31: Mountain below Stream is called *Xián* 咸 - "Mutual harmonious influence" and Hexagram 32: Wind below Thunder is called *Héng* 恆 "Long-lasting." On one level, both of these hexagrams refer to intimate relationships in marriage. Adapted from translation by Taoist Master Alfred Huang (1998). *The Complete I-Ching: The Definitive Translation*, p. 272.

[115] Following some Confucian traditions, Professor Cheng chooses to number the offspring 1-6 that are born to the two parents Heaven and Earth.

[116] There is another arrangement known as the Later Heaven or postnatal arrangement (*hòutiān* 後天) that some scholars believe shifts the trigrams to be in accord with the practical *yīnyáng–wǔxíng* 陰陽五行 (*yīnyáng* & Five Phase) dynamics. This arrangement is traditionally attributed to King Wen of Zhou (Zhōu Wénwáng 周文王; 1152-1050 BCE), who was considered by Confucius to be the paragon of the Sage King (*shèng wáng* 聖王). This Later Heaven arrangement has its origins in the *Luòshū* 洛書 (*Luo River Writing*) and creates what is known as the Magic Square seen in Figure 4.

Chapter 4: Hún and Pò 魂魄[117]

Lǎozǐ 老子 says:

載營魄抱一能無離乎

"Can one unify the spirit of the blood and the spirit of the breath and keep them from separating?"[118]

The *Nèijīng* 《內經》*(Internal Medicine Classic)* refers to *yíng* 營 and *wèi* 衛.[119] *Yíng* corresponds to the blood and *wèi* corresponds to the breath. So what is said (by Lǎozǐ) to be *yíng* and *pò* is the same as *hún* 魂 and *pò* 魄 because *hún* is associated with the movement of blood and *pò* is associated with the movement of breath or "warming *qì*" (*rè qì* 热氣).[120]

In the living body, blood *qì* is considered heavy (*yīn*) and tends to flow down (with gravity) while breath *qì* ("warming *qì*"), which is light, tends to flow up (and out) (and therefore more *yáng* by nature). At death, when blood and breath are no longer integrated, their *qì* movements reverse direction. This is why it is said in the classics that at death the *hún* (associated with the spirits of blood) fly *upward (evaporate)* and the *pò* (associated with the spirits of breath *qì*) descend.[121]

陽之精氣曰神，陰之精氣曰靈

Zéngzi[122] said "the essence of *qì* of *yáng* is called *shén*, [which is associated with the warming *qì* of breath]. The essence *qì* of *yīn* is called *líng* [which is called the *qì* of blood.]"[123]

The *yīn-yáng* relationship between *líng* and *shén* respectively corresponds to that between *hún* and *pò*. When the *hún* and *pò* are separated (at death), so too do *shén* and *líng* leave the body.[124] In cases where *shén* and *líng* depart but *hún* and *pò* do not, this is called a "ghost" (*guǐ* 鬼) that exists without a physical body or consciousness.[125] I don't know how Westerners will interpret *hún* and *pò* theory; since ghosts cannot be detected by the human eye or Western technology, they are viewed with suspicion and doubt.

To Western doctors, this may seem to have no practical usefulness or meaning because only the essence and blood belong to matter; matter (mass) is thought to never be destroyed.[126] Not only does East Asian medicine speak of the indestructibility of matter, but it also has its own terms regarding transformation of matter to offer to the doctors and philosophers of the West to investigate in detail.[127] While the separation of *hún* and *pò* at death may be of limited use to Western doctors, their importance in terms of function when united cannot be overstated. I hope the contemporary medical world will take notice of this.[128]

Arrangement of Terminology Used by the Sages[129]

Lǎozǐ 老子	***Nèijīng* 內經**	**Zēngzǐ 曾子**	**Designation**	***Qì* type**
Yíng 營 (Hún 魂)	Yíng 營	Líng 靈	Yīn 陰	Xuè qì 血氣 (blood/*qì*)
Pò 魄	Wèi 衛	Shén 神	Yáng 陽	Rè qì 熱氣 (warming breath *qì*)

Ch. 4 Notes

---

117 *Hún* 魂 represents "spiritual vigor." The classics say it is housed in the Liver and is associated with a kind of spirit-consciousness associated with forward thinking, planning ahead. The ideogram shows an image of a cloud-ghost-spirit often referred to as "ethereal soul" that comes and goes depending on our level of wakefulness. *Hún* being associated with the Liver has a relationship to the movement of blood circulation. It was perhaps this evolutionary development that enabled neolithic peoples to visualize the future, and put food away in their caves in order to survive the last ice age!

Pò 魄 represents "physical vigor." It is said to be housed in the Lung. The ideogram shows a white/clear-ghost-spirit often referred to as the "corporeal soul." It is said to "open and close" in accordance with breath. Like the pairs: *yīn-yáng*, *hún-pò* makes a coupled unit commonly translated as "soul" whose whole is greater than the sum of the parts. When breath and blood circulate together, we have a felt sense of physical and mental vigor." (from Cowan & Rosenberg (2025), *A Ring Without End:Reflections on Classical Chinese Medicine Mind/body Mapping.* See Appendix III: *Etymological Glossary of Sage Principle Terms,* for a more detailed analysis of these characters.

118 This quote is from the first line of Lǎozǐ 10 from *Lao-Tzu: My Words Are Very Easy to Understand. Lectures on the Tao Teh Ching:* Cheng & Gibbs (1981),p. 46.

119 In East Asian medicine, *yíng* 營 literally translated as "camp" refers to "nutritive *qì*," which is said to be the nourishing aspects of blood that flows in the blood vessels and irrigates the tissues of the body. In classical Chinese medicine both blood and hun have a close correspondence with the Liver (Wood element). *Wèi* 衛 (literally translated as "guard") refers to defensive or immune protective functions in the body. It is associated with the Lung (Metal element) which is said to house the *pò* 魄 (corporeal soul/spirit). *Hún* 魂 (ethereal soul/spirit) also corresponds to the spirit of dreams and *pò* to the spirit of the bones. Here Professor Cheng is making a uniquely original point of using the Lǎozi text to understand the dynamic *yīn-yáng* relationship between what he's calling "the spirit of the blood" and "the spirit of the breath," which in medicine, corresponds to the *yīn-yáng* interrelationship: *yīn* (*yíng qì* 營氣 and *hún* 魂) and *yáng* (*wèi qì* 衛氣 and *pò* 魄).

120 "Warming *qì*" (*rè qì* 热氣) literal translation: "steaming." Here Professor Cheng has chosen an old Daoist medical term to refer to the natural metabolic warmth generated in the body akin to the physiological warming effects of breathing (as in warming one's hands by breathing on them, or the effect of sunlight on our skin). This should be differentiated from pathological forms of Heat *yán*炎 (as in inflammation).

121 Here Professor Cheng explains the process of separation of *yīn-yáng* that takes place at death. In East Asian medical texts, it is said that *hún* and *pò* are no longer bound to each other. The *hún* (cloud spirits) fly off into the sky, leaving the *pò* (white spirits) as remains (bleached bones) in the ground. Thus *yīn-yáng* aspects of our soul/spirit separate and reverse direction: *yīn* (*hún*) which is usually heavy, now dissipates upward and *yáng* (*pò*) which is usually light, now is buried.

122 Zēngzǐ 曾子 (Tseng-tzu), also called Zēngcán (505-436 BCE), was a Chinese philosopher, disciple of Confucius and revered as one of the four sages of Confucianism, believed by some to be one of the authors of the "Great Learning" (Dà Xué 大學). Here Professor Cheng is again relating the principles of the Sages to the system of medicine.

123 Professor Cheng now further extends the correspondence between *yīn-yáng*, (*hún* and *pò*, blood and breath) to include the two kinds of animations (*qì*) that come from breath (*rèqì*) and blood (*xuèqì*). He makes a correspondence with spiritual/consciousness terms, *shén* 神 and *líng* 靈, in order to explain the meaning of a ghost that persists after a person dies, which he says is a disembodied spirit, a concept that may lie beyond the scope of most Western doctors.

Shén 神 and *líng* 靈 are complex psycho-spiritual terms mentioned in both Daoist and Confucian sage texts. *Shénlíng* as a couple means "Spirit" or spiritual power." *Shén,* often translated as spirit, relates to the states of consciousness, wakefulness, awareness and charisma while *líng* has many meanings depending on context, translated as spirited, lively, clever, quick, alert, efficacious. Professor Cheng is pointing out another important *yīn-yáng* relationship between *shén* and *líng* as aspects of consciousness/awareness and intelligence that have a correspondence with the soul/spirits of *hún* and *pò*.

124 When *shén* 神 and *líng* 靈 leave the body, it implies that there is no more consciousness.

125 Note that both *hún* 魂 and *pò* 魄 characters contain the *guǐ* 鬼 ghost radical within them. See Appendix III: *Etymological Glossary of Sage Principle Terms*, for a more detailed analysis of these characters.

126 The Law of Conservation of Mass dates from Antoine Lavoisier's 1789 discovery that mass is neither created nor destroyed in chemical reactions. In other words, the mass of any one element at the beginning of a reaction will equal the mass of that element at the end of the reaction.

127 The law of conservation of mass is defined in terms of closed systems of matter. Professor Cheng is perhaps suggesting here that the East Asian medicine's perspective views any part as a microcosm of the whole, in a state of constant flux that reflects the whole and thus cannot be considered a closed system.

---

128 Professor Cheng is making a direct point to Western medical practitioners to consider the importance of *yīn-yáng* dynamic unity and the inseparability of mind-body-spirit in promoting health.

129 Professor Cheng has created an innovative chart that correlates the terminology of the sages (Lǎozi and Zēngzǐ) with the classical medical terms (*Huáng Dì Nèijīng* 《黃帝內經》) as they correspond to *yīn-yáng* pairs: different names for the same relationships.

Chapter 5: Essence-Spirit and Blood-Breath Jīngshén Xuèqì 精神血氣[130]

Explanation Concerning Refinement of Essence (*jīng* 精) into Vital Essence-Breath (*jīngqì*).

According to the Internal Medicine Classic, "The Kidneys (genitourinary organ network) rule the Water; they receive the essence (*jīng*) from the five organs and six viscera (*zàngfǔ*),[131] and they store it (as seminal fluids).[132] According to Western medicine, one drop of seminal fluid is as precious as forty drops of blood.[133] According to East Asian medicine, during sexual intercourse, when men and women first produce *jīng*-essence, it must pass through the "sea of *qì*" or *dāntián* 丹田,[134] coming down through the "origin pass" (*guānyuán* 關源)[135] before emerging.[136] If sexual behavior is unrestrained, the *jīng* (essence) drains out and is lost. In Chinese, to say that someone is promiscuous is to call them "downward drained," meaning "vulgar."[137] Sages like Emperor Huángdì and Lǎozǐ not only practiced sexual self-restraint, but also utilized these fluids for the cultivation of health and longevity. This method is called *liànjīng* 煉精 or "distillation of seminal essence fluid."[138] To distill or refine the essence-fluids into "vital essence-breath" (*jīngqì* 精氣) (also called "procreative *qì*") is the first and foremost step in the discipline and practice of Chinese Sage Cultivation Principles.[139]

This may be explained as follows: The refining of essence fluids (*jīng*) can enhance spirit-consciousness (*shén*), and this is something that anyone can achieve, though all too often excessive sexual behavior results in loss of this ability. Emperor

Huang and Lǎozǐ were considered the pioneers at mastering this self-cultivation method, known as the "technique of refining essence and transforming *qì*."[140] The main focus of practice concerns the *dāntián.*

Dāntián 丹田 or "Sea of Qì" (*qìhǎi* 氣海), is also referred to as "the chamber of hidden essence."[141] *Dāntián* literally means the "field" (*tián* 田) for refining "elixir" (*dān* 丹).[142] Its location is in the abdomen, one and three-tenths of an inch (*cùn* 寸) below the navel, closer inside to the front of the abdomen than to the spine in the proportion: three-tenths from the front, seven-tenths from the back.

Concentrating the Heart/mind[143] and the (breath-*qì*) together in the *dāntián* means nourishing *jīng* by the warming vital *qì* (*rèqì* 熱氣) of blood circulation (*xuèqì*). The spirit (*shén*) of the Heart-mind (*xīn*) continues to be focused firmly there. By breathing in the air (*tiānqì* 天氣), it continues to be directed towards the *dāntián*, allowing the essence (*jīng*) that passes through the *dāntián* to be retained and activated there. By diligently concentrating the Heart/mind and breath-*qì* together there, over time, the essence (*jīng*) can be warmed,[144] transforming into a kind of heat (*rèlì* 熱力)[145] akin to electrical power (*diànlì*)[146] which can soak into the membranes, sinews and ligaments of the tailbone and sacrum, entering the spaces between the joints.[147] This refined essence (*liànjīng* 煉精) then enters the inside of the bones of the sacrum (and lower spine) where it cools, condensing into a thin mist like sweat that coats the interior walls of the bones where, with further cooling, it solidifies into marrow.[148] When the bones are enriched with this ripening marrow, it will eventually extend up the spine to the brain, which is called the "sea of marrow" (*suǐ hǎi* 髓海) in East Asian medicine.[149] This, then, is what is known as the method of refining *jīng* essence (*liànjīng* 煉精)."

Ch. 5 Notes

---

130 *Jīng* 精 (essence), *shén* 神 (spirit), *xuè* 血 (blood), *qì* 氣 (vital force). *Jīng* 精, is defined by Ames & Hall (2003) as "potency" and represents the essential material form of life, associated with sperm or ovum. *Jīngqì* 精氣 discussed later in this chapter is the procreative energy that drives vitality and arousal. As mentioned in *Lǎozǐ* 55, *Jīng* 精 describes the virtues of a newborn: "*Though his bones are soft and sinews supple, his grip is firm. As yet oblivious to the copulation of male and female, his member still stands erect. Such is the height of potency (extreme jīng),*" Ames & Hall (2003), p. 163. *Shén* 神 ("spirit") represents consciousness or the spiritual aspect of being alive, intimately connected to *jīng*. Likewise, *xuè* 血 (blood) and *qì* 氣 (vital breath) are paired, complementary forces: blood provides substance, while *qì* activates circulation. (See *Arrangement of Terminology Used by the Sages* in the previous chapter, p. 60). Classical Chinese medicine holds that "the blood carries the *qì*, and the *qì* moves the blood." Together, *jīng/shén* and *xuè/qì* illustrate the interdependence of material and immaterial aspects of life, a principle central to both *tàijí* practice and East Asian medicine. See Appendix III: *Etymological Glossary of Sage Principle Terms*, for a more detailed analysis of these characters.

131 *Zàngfǔ* 臟 腑 translated as "organs and viscera" refer to the five solid (*yīn*) *zàng* organs and the six hollow (*yáng*) *fǔ* viscera. The five *zàng* organs are Liver, Heart, Spleen, Lung, Kidney that correspond to the five phases/elements: Wood, Fire, Earth, Metal, Water, respectively. The six *fǔ* viscera are: Gall Bladder, Small Intestine, Stomach, Large Intestine, Bladder plus the Triple Warmer (*Sān jiāo* 三膲).

132 *Huáng Dì Nèijīng Sùwèn* 《黃帝內經素問》 Chapter 1, *Jīng* 精 here means male and female seminal fluids which are thought to be distilled from the secretions of the other organs. Unschuld & Tessenow (2011), p. 40

133 I'm not sure where Professor Cheng is getting this statistic in Western medicine, but he seems to be suggesting that the loss of essence-fluids should be guarded as carefully as one would with the loss of blood.

134 "Sea of Qì"(*Qìhǎi* 氣海) refers to acupuncture point *Rén* 6 on the abdomen approximately 1.5 inches below the umbilicus and is considered the access point to the *dāntián* 丹田. (See Chapter 9 for further discussion of the *dāntián.*)

135 *Guānyuán* 關源 (Kwan Yuan) "Origin Pass" refers to the important acupuncture point *Rén* 4 on the midline of the abdomen approximately 2 inches above the pubic symphysis. It is a tonifying point used in many urinary and gynecological conditions.

136 This refers to the male and female fluids produced by the genitalia.

[137] Xiàliú 下流 literally "low-flowing", meaning "vulgar, obscene, low class." In Chapter 1 of the *Huáng Dì Nèijīng Sùwèn* 《黃帝內經素問》 Unschuld & Tessenow (2011), p. 32, refers to this *"The fact that people of today are different is because, they take wine as an [ordinary] beverage, and they adopt absurd [behavior] as regular [behavior]. They are drunk when they enter the [women's] chambers. Through their lust, they exhaust their essence, through their wastefulness they dissipate their true [qi]."*

Wáng Bì 王弼 makes a note to clarify this in his commentary: *"If one takes pleasure in sex without limits, then one's essence will be exhausted. If one makes frivolous use [of one's essence] without end, then the true qi will be dissipated. Hence it is because the sages cherished [their] essence and carefully considered its use that their bones were full of marrow and strong. Lǎozǐ has said: '[The sages] weaken their wills (desires) and strengthen their bones."* ibid. pp. 32-33.

[138] *Liàn* 煉 (*làn*, lien) translates as "to smelt;" "refine;" "distill."*Liàn jīng* 煉精 is a term referring to the Daoist alchemy practices called "Refinement of Essential Matter into Vital Breath" (*liànjīng huàqì* 煉精化氣) expounded by such masters as Zhāng Zǐyáng 張紫陽 during the Song dynasty.

Daniel Schrier, editor: An essential dimensions of Daoist practice-realization, is *xiūliàn* 修煉/修鍊 (cultivation-and-refinement). It may be understood as shorthand for *xiūdào* 修道 (cultivating the Dao) and *liàndān* 煉丹 (refining the elixir), reflecting both agricultural and alchemical metaphors of growth, transformation, and transmutation. The character *xiū* 修 conveys cultivation and self-development, while *liàn* 煉/鍊 implies refining through fire or metalwork, symbolizing the transformative process of practice. In Daoist cultivation traditions, *xiūliàn* frequently refers to practices of internal alchemy (*nèidān* 內丹), focusing on the refinement of body (*xíng* 形) and qì through disciplined practice, meditation, and energetic transformation. Related terms include *xiūxíng* 修行 (cultivation and practice) and *xiūzhēn* 修真, (cultivating the "Real" or "Perfection").

Towards the end of the Tang and beginning of the Song, internal alchemy (*nèidān*) also referred to as the "Golden Elixir" (*jīndān* 金丹) became more systematized. These practices employ symbolic language to describe psychosomatic refinement, and transforming the human body into a cosmological or spiritual entity. The goal being "immortality" or "transcendence," which is achieved through energetic transformations that generate the "immortal embryo" (*xiāntāi* 仙胎) and the "yang-spirit" (*yángshén*陽神). Central to this tradition are the internal Three Treasures (*nèi sānbǎo*內三寶): vital essence (*jīng* 精), subtle breath (*qì* 氣), and spirit (*shén*神), which are refined through a three-stage process: 1) refining vital essence into qi (*liàn jīng huà qì*煉精化氣), 2) refining qi into spirit (*liàn qì huà shén*煉氣化神), and 3) refining spirit to return to Emptiness (*liàn shén huán xū* 煉神還虛). This framework underlies classical internal alchemy, linking bodily cultivation with cosmological and spiritual transcendence.

139 Qì 炁 this is an early symbol for *qì* 氣 used specifically by Daoists in their alchemical practices. The ideogram contains the symbol for inhaling or swallowing placed above the fire symbol. In choosing this character, Professor Cheng is differentiating this form of *qì* from the general term for *qì* 氣 (breath) to indicate its "vital procreative force," and though we have no easy translation of the ideogram 炁 we might call it "esoteric breath" or "procreative *qì*." See Appendix III: *Etymological Glossary of Sage Principle Terms*, for a more detailed analysis of these characters.

140 "Technique of refining essence and transforming *qì*" (*jiàn jīnghuà zěn zhīfǎ* 鍊精化怎之法).

141 "Chamber for storing hidden essence" (*cáng jīng zhī shì* 藏精之室).

142 *Dāntián* 丹田 (tan-t'ien) see Chapter 9 for further discussion.

143 It is important to remember that *xīn* 心 carries the double meaning of both "mind" and " Heart" in East Asian medicine and is likened to the Emperor of organs in charge of circulating *shén* 神 "consciousness" throughout the body by way of the blood, the so-called "distributed mind."

144 In East Asian medicine and Daoist practice, *nuǎn* 暖 ("to warm") often refers to the promotion of heat and circulation in the body to support vitality, proper organ function, and the movement of *qì* 氣.

145 *Rèlì* 熱力 ("to heat up") refers to the active generation or presence of heat/energy, often in the context of the warmth of the body, by way of *qì* circulation, or metabolic energetic processes.

146 *Diàn lì* 電力 *("electrical power") diàn* 電 is also the character for lightning, reflecting the natural phenomenon from which the concept of electricity is derived. *Lì* means "force" or "power," so *diànlì* literally conveys the idea of the power of lightning.

147 It's interesting to note that Western scientific research has recently discovered a "new" organ called "the interstitium" that is composed of spaces within the connective tissue that extends throughout the body and is physiologically active, being circulated not by the Heart but by way of the movement of muscles and tendons. See Chapter 6 for more on the interstitium and Benias & Thiess, (2018). *The New Tissue That Could Change Medicine.*

148 *Sui* 髓 (Marrow): There is some interesting recent Western medical research evidence that hemopoietic (blood forming) stem cells are located in close proximity to the thin layer of cells of the inner lining of bone endosteum. These multi-potential stem cells can transform into any type of blood cell in the body. See Zhang, et al. (2007). *Hematopoietic Stem Cells with Higher Hematopoietic Potential Reside at the Bone Marrow Endosteum.*

149 *Suǐhǎi* 髓海 (Sea of marrow) in classical Chinese medicine, refers to the brain tissue, which is considered one of the six "curious organs" (*qíhéng zhī fǔ* 奇恒之腑) (also called the "extraordinary organs") that include: brain, marrow, bones, blood vessels, gallbladder and uterus. The relationship between marrow and brain is like that of streams flowing to the sea, as Elizabeth Rochat states: "*One of the differences between the brain and marrow is that the brain is like a sea, immobile and fixed…but what flows into the sea is circulating and this is the marrow…one of the main functions of the marrow is to circulate and irrigate, to flow into the bones, the skull, the hollows and the orifices. This is the movement inside the bones. The bones are like the riverbed, the stones and the rocks of the earth.*" Larre & Rochat de la Vallée (2003). *The Extraordinary Fu*, p. 93.

Chapter 6: The System of Tendons, Channels, and Membrane Networks 筋脈与膜膈之系统[150]

East Asian medicine recognizes the system of *qì* circulation and places emphasis on four parts of the body where this circulation takes place: tendons, channels, membranes and the diaphragm. The principal theories of meridian-channels and membranes mainly refer to the two aspects that Western medicine has not paid attention to, which can be summarized in one word: *qì*. What is referred to as *qì* is the motive force of blood circulation; if we do not speak of *qì*, then the circulation of blood loses its active function, which is problematic.[151]

In the practice of *tàijí quán* 太极拳 *(t'ai chi ch'üan)*, one earnestly seeks relaxation and resiliency in order to accentuate the functional circulation of blood-*qì*. Therefore, by sinking the breath/*qì* down to the *dāntián*, it is mobilized by the membranes and diaphragm, communicating with the sinews/tendons which causes the channels to flow. This not only facilitates blood circulation, but also allows the five organs and six bowels (*zàngfǔ* 臟腑), and various other parts of the body, to achieve comfortable movement through the harmonious interaction of blood and *qì*.[152]

According to the language of Western medical embryology, the primary "lumen"[153] is the space in the blastocyst[154] (see Figure 17).

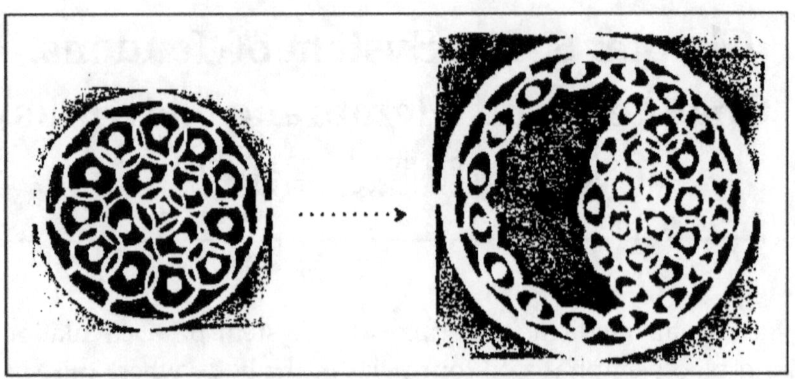

Figure 17: Formation of the Blastocoel and Inner Cell Mass
Illustration by Ed Young[155]

As the blastocyst develops into the embryo, the lumen (blastocoel) gradually reduces in size until it seems to be lost. In East Asian medicine, this "primordial *lú-mén*" is called the "Sea of Qì" (*qìhǎi* 氣海),[156] also referred to as the *dāntián*. It is related to what Western medicine calls the "Greater Omentum."[157] This primordial *lú-mén* is the center of the body's system of membranes and interstitial spaces.[158] There is no part of the body, including the skin, that does not depend upon the functional flow of *qì* from the diaphragm through the membranes. Its origin is indeed in the *dāntián*.

Ch. 6 Notes

---

150 *Jīnmài* 筋脈 refers to the integrated system of tendons and sinews (*jīn* 筋) and vessels or channels (*mài* 脈). *Mógé* 膜膈 denotes membranous networks, with *mó* 膜 meaning membrane and *gé* 膈 referring anatomically to the diaphragm, a large musculotendinous structure enveloped in fascia that spans the thoracic and abdominal cavities. The rhythmic movement of the diaphragm during respiration promotes circulation and continuity within these interconnected membranous pathways, reflecting the *tàijí* 太極 principle that "when one part moves, all parts move." Contemporary physiology further recognizes the diaphragm as a multifunctional structure involved not only in respiration but also in venous and lymphatic return, modulation of cardiac hemodynamics and autonomic tone, lumbar spine stabilization and postural control, lymph drainage from the thorax and upper extremities, and gastroesophageal functions including swallowing and reflux regulation. See Powers (2025). *Diaphragm Function in Health and Disease.*

151 The Chinese medical classics emphasize the interdependent relationship between blood and *qì*. As noted in the previous chapter, *"qì moves the blood, and blood carries the qì,"* much like a mother nurturing her child. In this sense, the blood– *qì* pair (*xuèqì* 血氣) represents a fundamental embodiment of the *yīn-yáng* principle (see chart in Chapter 4).

152 In reference to improving blood circulation, recent research has demonstrated that *Tàijí quán* may be beneficial in reducing blood pressure. See Yeh, et al. (2008), *The Effect of Tai Chi Exercise on Blood Pressure.*

153 Professor Cheng employed a transliterated rendering of the Western term *"lumen"* as *lú-mén* 廬門 (literally "secret door"). Notably, this choice also preserves the semantic sense of the original term: *lú* denotes a corridor or passageway, while *mén* refers to a gate or portal, together evoking the idea of an internal channel or opening.

154 It is interesting to note that Professor Cheng closely examined evidence from modern cell biology and sought to correlate these findings with East Asian medicine and Daoist practice. During embryonic development, cells undergo rapid division and become increasingly compact, with the cytoplasm subdivided at each successive division. Toward the end of the approximately five-day period, a cavity begins to form within the cellular mass, giving rise to the hollow blastocyst. The blastocyst consists of roughly 150 cells arranged as a sphere, comprising an outer cellular layer (the trophoblast), a fluid-filled cavity (the blastocoel), and an internal cluster of cells known as the inner cell mass.

155 Illustration by Ed Young depicts the progression of multiplication of embryonic cells to create an open cavity (blastocoel) that will eventually become the yolk sac as the inner cell mass becomes the embryo. This is based on original drawings from *Cunningham's Textbook of Anatomy* that Professor Cheng was apparently examining during the writing of this book.

---

156 *Qìhǎi* 氣海 noted in the previous chapter is the name for the acupuncture point Ren 6 that lies 1.5 cm below the umbilicus that serves as a gateway giving access to the *dāntián* 丹田.

157 Omentum: *wǎng mó* 网膜 (*wǎng* 网 – "network" and *mó* 膜 – "membranes") Professor Cheng was studying the anatomy of membrane networks including the organ-structure known as the omentum, and had developed a radical theory that this is where the *dāntián* is located and how it functions in moving blood/*qì* through the body. Professor Cheng is proposing here that the embryonic cavity which eventually devolves is actually the functional center of this system of membrane networks. He emphasized the importance of subtle circulation within these membrane networks which has gone unnoticed by Western medicine until only recently when it was recognized as a distinct "organ" now dubbed the "Interstitium." *"The interstitium is a body-wide network of fluid-filled spaces within connective tissue that acts as a "shock absorber" and a transport system. Once thought to be dense structural tissue, recent research using new microscopy techniques has revealed it as a connected, fluid-filled mesh that surrounds organs, nerves, and vessels."* (See Benias, et al. (2018), *Structure and Distribution of an Unrecognized Interstitium in Human Tissues.)*

158 The omentum is an abdominal membranous sac (bursa) contained by aspects of the central mesenteric ligaments. See Chapter 9 *Dāntián* 丹田 for more in-depth discussion on the relationship between *dāntián* and Omentum.

PART II[159]

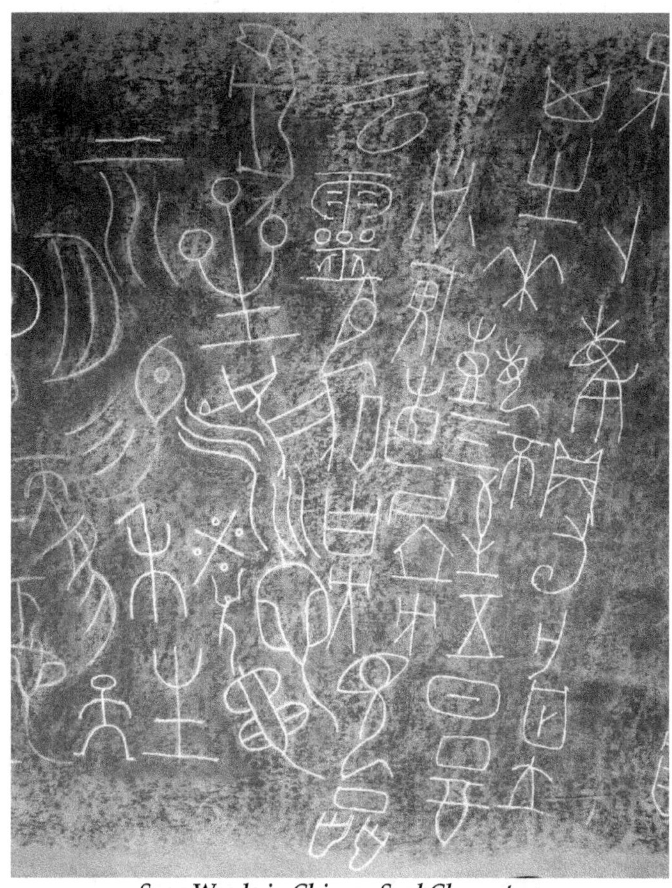

Sage Words in Chinese Seal Characters
created by Ed Young

[159] Note: Professor Cheng has organized this book to reflect his integrative way of thinking in such a way as to help guide the student in making corresponding connections. In the same way that the *Yìjīng* 《易經》 64 hexagrams are divided into two parts: Hexagrams 1-31 are said to represent the Dao of Heaven and Earth and hexagrams 32-64 are said to represent the Dao of Humanity, in this book, Part I presents the big macro-cosmological Sage Principles of *yīn-yáng* 陰陽 and the *bāguà* 八卦 (eight trigrams), including our spirit/consciousness connection to the Heavens and Earth (*hún* 魂, *pò* 魄, *jīng*精, *qì* 氣, *shén* 神) extending down to the physical level of blood vessels and tendons, all the way to the embryonic beginnings of a human being. Part II explores the microcosmic examination of specific aspects of human life that is the foundation of East Asian medicine, beginning with the five phase (*wǔxíng* 五行) relations of the organs. In so doing, Professor Cheng demonstrates how the words of the Sages apply to our personal health and daily life.

Chapter 7: Yīn-Yáng, Five Phases and the Five Organs 陰陽五行五臟[160]

Yīn-yáng and the Five Phases (*wǔ xíng* 五行) are the Sage Principles scientific studies[161] that differentiate Eastern and Western thought. However, the concepts of *yīn-yáng*, as well as their interactions, are relevant to the philosophy and science of the West, but there exists a gap in understanding. It is a pity that many people in the West have not yet grasped the significance of these concepts, which is why I will elaborate on their roles as well as the polarity present in all of Nature – such as male/female, hot/cold, dry/wet, hard/soft etc. All things in nature can be understood in terms of having properties of *yīn-yáng*.

Within the Chinese Sage Principles, these concepts form a fundamental key to polarity, much the way modern physicists analyze the atomic structures of matter down to the point that they cannot be further divided; yet even at that extreme, there still seem to exist two types of divergent properties (positive and negative charges) that are in many ways akin to the concept of *yīn-yáng*. For example, when one transmits radio waves, though it can be said that they are invisible to the naked eye, they are nevertheless produced by the oscillation between (+) and (-) charged poles similar to the movement of *yīn-yáng*.[162]

Five thousand years ago, Fú Xī 伏羲 created the 64 Hexagrams, based on the ancient He-River Diagram and Luo Writing which illustrated this same *yīn-yáng* dynamic. To clarify its principles, Confucius expanded on the *Book of Changes* with his commentaries. That text discusses the origins of the

River Luo and the necessity of a strong human presence to govern it.[163] It addresses the five phases: Metal, Wood, Water, Fire, and Soil/Earth, which are generated by the Heavens and Earth and possess interdependent properties. It also references the principles of the *Luò Shū* 《洛書》 writing that emphasize the foundational nature of these five phases in understanding the *Yìjīng* 《易經》 (*Book of Changes*). The Confucian commentaries highlight the interrelationships of the five phases and *yīn-yáng* dynamics, by explaining their individual properties. These Laws of Nature have scientific implications in comprehending all material existence.

The five phases are Metal, Water, Wood, Fire, and Soil/ Earth.[164] The relationships between these five involve cycles of mutual generation and control.[165]

The system of generation (*shēng* 生) is as follows:

1. Metal generates Water.[166] When metal is heated, it becomes a liquid. Likewise, a mountain of stone generates the streams.
2. Water generates Wood; plants naturally grow when watered, which is the essence of water giving rise to wood.[167]
3. Wood generates Fire. The ancients used to drill wood to make fire, which is the essence of how wood feeds fire.[168]
4. Fire generates Soil/Earth. The ashes and mulch of plants generate the soil.[169]
5. Earth generates Metal. All metals come from deep within the soil.

This cycle is the unending mutual generation of the five phases; the five act as friends helping each other in the succession of the seasons throughout the year, seen in Figure 18.

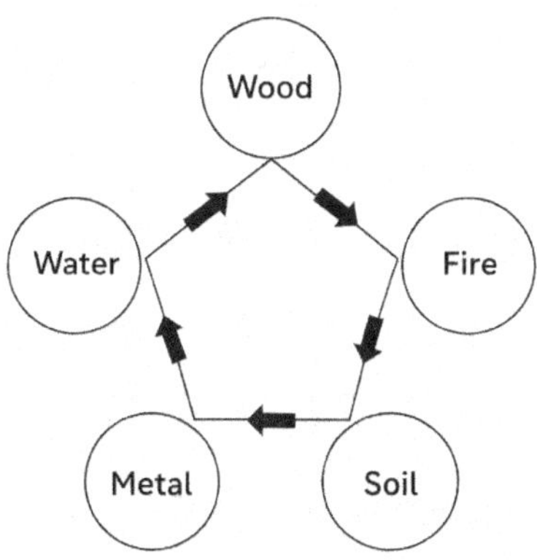

Figure 18: Shēng 生 Generating Cycle of Five Phases

The system of control (*kè* 剋) is as follows:

1. Metal can carve or cut down wood. This is the Metal spirit controlling Wood.
2. The roots of trees extend straight down into the soil. This is the Wood spirit having control over the Soil/Earth.
3. The soil can absorb water and can also channel water pathways. This is the Earth spirit controlling Water.
4. Water can suppress fire. This is the Water spirit overcoming Fire.
5. Fire can melt metal. This is the Fire spirit overcoming the hardness of Metal.

This is the system of the five elements overcoming one another seen in Figure 19.

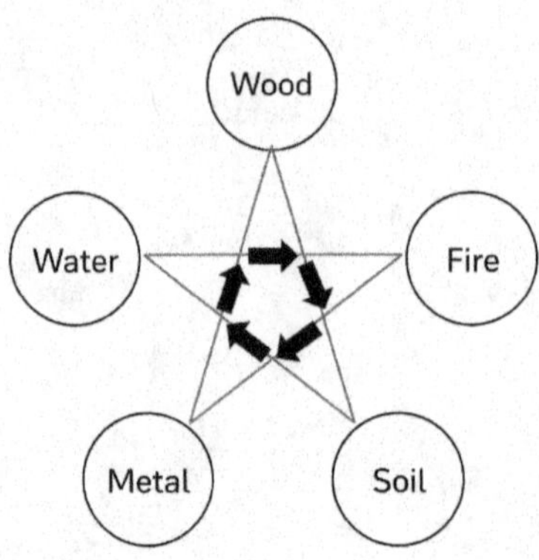

Figure 19: Kè 剋 Controlling Cycle of the Five phases

The Five Phases and the Five Zang Organs

The relationships of the five phases correspond to the five organs[170] and proceed in the same sequence of generative (*shēng* 生) and controlling (*kè* 剋) cycles. Details of the correspondences between the phases and the organ networks are stated in the *Internal Medicine Classic.*[171]

The Shēng - Generating Cycle of the Organ Networks

1. **The Lung** corresponds to the Metal phase: By absorbing air, the Lungs generate a liquid elixir[172] just as snow will condense at the top of a mountain of stone. This elixir sinks down into the Kidney (genitourinary/adrenal system), giving life to it and making it strong. So it is said that the Lungs are like the "mother"and the Kidney is like the "child" receiving nourishment in accordance with five phase *shēng* dynamics. East Asian medicine uses "Metal"

to designate Lungs for reasons of convenience and simplicity, just like the mathematician uses algebraic symbols to represent numerical concepts. It is therefore said that just as Metal generates Water, the Lungs nourish the Kidney, consistent with the generative principle of the five phases.[173]

2. **The Kidney** (urogenital/adrenal system) corresponds to the phase of Water. Water nourishes Wood (growth of vegetation). Likewise, the Kidneys are said to nourish the Liver which corresponds to the Wood phase.[174]

3. **The Liver** corresponds to the phase of Wood. In Nature, Wood feeds Fire. Fire corresponds to the Heart. The Liver functions as storage of blood and promotes blood flow to the Heart. Thus it is said that the Liver nourishes the Heart.[175]

4. **The Heart** corresponds to the Fire phase. In the process of burning, Fire makes ashes, which feed the Soil/Earth. Earth corresponds to the digestive system comprising the Spleen/Pancreas organ network. Therefore the Heart is said to nourish the Spleen (digestion).[176]

5. **The Spleen** corresponds to the elemental phase of Earth. Earth in turn gives rise to Metal; therefore, the Spleen (digestion) is said to nourish the Lungs.[177]

This relationship is known as the five organs nourishing one another according to the Five Phases they correspond to, as illustrated in Figure 20.

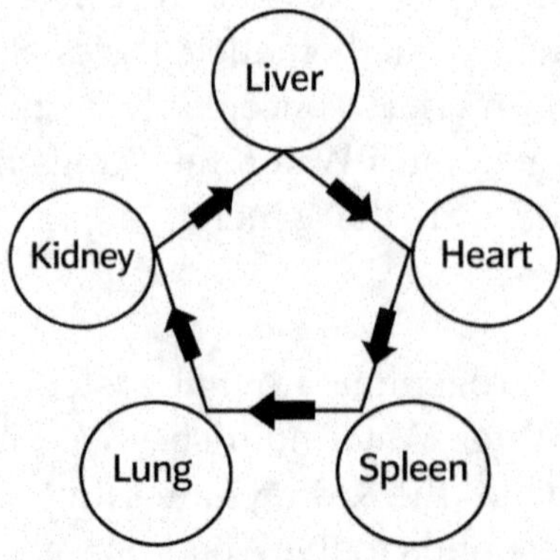

Figure 20: The Shēng /Generating Cycle of the Organ Networks

The Kè Cycle of Control of the Function of the Five Organs

When one organ is overloaded, it will affect the organ network that it controls or is controlled by it. For example:

1. The Lungs correspond to the Metal Phase, and Metal can cut down Wood. If one's Lungs are inflamed or congested, Liver functions (Wood) will invariably be compromised.[178]
2. The Liver corresponds to the Wood Phase. Just as Wood can drive through the Earth, Liver dysfunction can suppress the Spleen's digestive processes.[179]
3. The Spleen corresponds to the Earth phase. Just as the soil can block a stream's water flow, the Spleen can suppress Kidney function.[180]
4. The Kidneys correspond to the Water phase. Just as water can put out a fire, Kidney dysfunction can repress Heart function.[181]
5. The Heart corresponds to the Fire phase. Just as a fire can melt metal, the Heart, when overloaded, can suppress Lung function.[182]

This relationship is known as the five organs overcoming one another according to the Five Phases they correspond to, as illustrated in Figure 21.

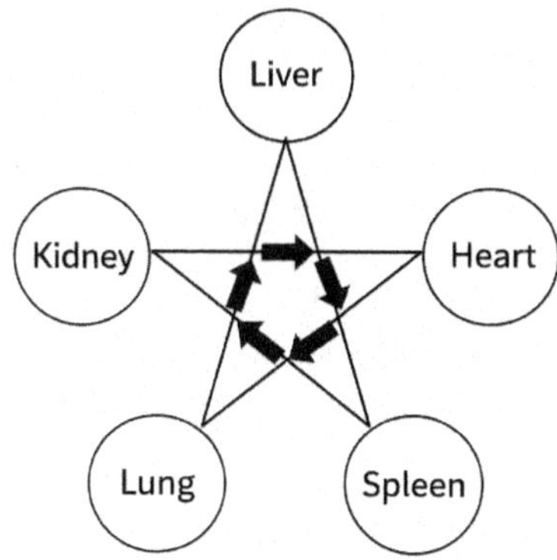

Figure 21: The Kè Controlling Cycle of the Organ Networks

Ch. 7 Notes

---

160 Five phases and five organs *wǔxíng wǔzàng* 五行五臟.

161 "Scientific" (*kēxué* 科学) the characters Professor Cheng is using for "science" is interesting: *kē* 科 means "department of science" and *xué* means "learning" or "knowledge." Together they imply the area of scientific knowledge or scientific study.

162 A radio transmitter applies oscillating electric current to the antenna, and the antenna radiates the power as radio waves. The oscillation occurs between (+) and (-) charged electrons.

163 The Luo River (*Luò Hé* 洛河) runs from Mount Huà (Huàshān 華山) and empties into the Yellow River. During the Warring States period (475-221 BCE) when Lăozi and Confucius lived, it was a contested site between the Qin and Wei states. The Luo River system, and its tributary, the Gu River, flowed through the heartland of multiple kingdoms, making its management crucial for imperial stability. This river system formed part of the complex hydrological network of ancient China's central plains, an area often called the cradle of Chinese civilization. This region, encompassing parts of modern Henan and Shaanxi provinces, was characterized by its fertile soil and numerous waterways that supported agricultural development and urban settlement.

164 Phase (*xíng* 行): The pictogram 行 depicts a pair of footprints, symbolizing movement. *Xíng* 行 conveys the idea of motion or activity and is commonly translated as to walk; to go; to travel; to circulate; to do; to perform; behavior; conduct. The common translation of *wŭxíng* 五行 as the "Five Elements" is technically misleading, as the term *xíng* emphasizes dynamic processes rather than static substances. Unlike the Western concept of an element, which is a fixed material entity, the five phases are better understood as five distinct movements, behaviors, or transformative processes observed in Nature. These five phases are: Earth/Soil (*tŭ* 土), Wood (*mù* 木), Water (*shuĭ* 水), Fire (*huŏ* 火), and Metal (*jīn* 金).

165 Generating (*shēng* 生) and Controlling (*kè* 剋/克): *Shēng* conveys the sense of "giving birth to" or "producing," while *kè* refers to "regulating;" "restraining;" or "controlling." See Appendix III: *Etymological Glossary of Sage Principle Terms*, for a more detailed analysis of these characters.

166 "Melting into water" in the system of correspondences presented in the *Huángdì Nèijīng*, Metal corresponds to Autumn and Water corresponds to Winter, thus Autumn gives rise to Winter.

167 In the system of correspondences presented in the *Huángdì Nèijīng*, Water corresponds to Winter and Wood corresponds to Spring, thus Winter gives rise to Spring.

168 In the system of correspondences presented in the *Huángdì Nèijīng*, Wood corresponds to Springtime and Fire to Summer, thus Spring gives rise to Summer.

169 The soil is a product of the rotting of plant material after it has ripened in harvest. In the *Luòshū* 洛書 and *Hétú* 河圖 diagrams of the *Yìjīng*, Earth/Soil (*tŭ* 土) is located at the center intersection of the four directions, representing the place that the four seasons revolve around. The ripening at the end of Summer gives rise to the harvest, that corresponds to the Soil/Earth phase in the five phases (*wŭxíng*) system.

[170] Organ (*zàng* 臟) - In contrast to the strictly anatomic designations of "organs" in Western medicine, East Asian medicine understands life as a system of correspondences. Within this framework, the "organs" (*zàng*) are conceived as networks of physiologic function within the body rather than just forms. This is the important relationship of *Lǐ–Qì–Xiàng* 理氣象, that Professor Cheng emphasized in Chapter 3.

For example, the "Lung organ network" refers to the respiratory and mucosal functions extending from the nostrils down through the respiratory tree and into the Lung, but also includes the middle ear and the sinuses as well as the skin. The "Kidney organ network" includes the urinary, reproductive (genital) and adrenal functions as well as the bone and marrow. The "Liver organ network" refers to the Liver's blood storing and processing function as well as the tendons and ligaments and some parts of the nervous system. The " Heart organ network" includes the circulatory system as well as the functional seat of emotions and consciousness. The "Spleen organ network" comprises the digestive processing as well as aspects of thought.

[171] *Huángdì Nèijīng Sùwèn,* Chapter 25 describes in great detail the relationships between the five phases (*wǔxíng* 五行). In the systematic correspondences: Wood corresponds with the Liver organ network, Fire with the Heart network, Earth with the Spleen network, Metal with the Lung network and Water with the Kidney network. A number of other chapters of the *Internal Medicine Classic* (*Huángdì Nèijīng*) further elaborate how disease patterns manifest in this systems-based medical model.

[172] The idea of the Lung producing a liquid or elixir may refer to what Professor Cheng mentioned in Chapter 5 regarding breathing into the *dāntián* to activate the *jīng* fluids and thereby creating *jīngqì* elixir. On the other hand, this may also refer to the relationship between *xuè* 血 (blood) and *qì* 氣 (air) mentioned in Chapter 4 in connection with *hún* 魂 and *pò* 魄. From a Western physiological perspective, one might draw a parallel with pulmonary respiration, in which the oxygenation of blood during inspiration transforms the blood (liquid) into a special activated (oxygenated) elixir that brings life to the body. However, it is important not to take this analogy too literally. East Asian medicine uses analogic terminology in its metaphor-based correspondences whereas Western medical terminology is based primarily on *analytic* reductive reasoning.

[173] "Generating" or "engendering" refers to *shēng* 生 the life-giving cycle of birth and growth in East Asian medicine. See Appendix III: *Etymological Glossary of Sage Principle Terms,* for a more detailed analysis of these characters.

[174] *"The Kidneys are said to nourish the Liver which corresponds to the Wood phase."* In Western medicine, the Kidney produces erythropoietin, a hormone that stimulates the production of red blood cells. The Liver in East Asian medicine is said to be in charge of storing the blood. Additionally, the Kidney produces the hormone Renin that is key in regulating blood pressure. In East Asian medicine, high blood pressure is typically understood to be related to the Kidney-Liver relationship. However, as previously stated, we must be cautious in making too literal a comparison between East Asian medicine and Western medicine, which runs the risk of dumbing down both medicines! Nevertheless, it is easy to imagine that Professor Cheng would have been thrilled to see the two systems of medicine engaging in dialogue and mutually informing one another.

[175] *"The Liver nourishes the Heart"* - There is research demonstrating the relationship between Liver and Heart function. For example, chronic Liver conditions such as cirrhosis can result in hepatic cardiomyopathy, illustrating a biomedical influence between hepatic and cardiac physiology. This relationship has been characterized in modern biomedical literature by Hadi et al. (2020) as a "two-way street" between Heart and Liver disease.

[176] *"The Heart nourishes the Spleen"* - In East Asian medicine, the Spleen, Stomach, duodenum and pancreas are considered components of the Earth digestive system. There is a large body of modern research demonstrating strong connections between nutrition and cardiovascular health, and conditions such as Heart failure can directly and indirectly impair digestion, absorption, and overall nutritional status.

[177] *"The Spleen nourishes the Lungs."* - In East Asian medicine, the Spleen's role in digestion and nutrient transformation underpins the production of *qì* that supports Lung function. Correspondingly, modern research has demonstrated significant relationships between nutritional status and respiratory health, with diet influencing Lung development, immune defense, and pulmonary function. See Berthon & Wood (2015), *Nutrition and Respiratory Health—Feature Review.*

[178] *The Lung affects Liver function.* It is well known that pulmonary conditions such as pneumonias can cause alterations in Liver function tests. This relationship was first documented and has since been observed in a wide range of pulmonary conditions, including COVID-19. See Capdevila et al. (1990). *Liver Alterations in Acute Pneumonia.*

[179] The Liver plays a central role in digestion, nutrient metabolism, and detoxification, contributing significantly to the breakdown of food, the absorption of nutrients, and the processing of metabolic byproducts. See Trefts, Gannon, & Wasserman (2017), *The Liver.*

---

180 *The Spleen (digestion) can block Kidney function.* For example, it is well known that disorders of digestive system such as constipation can disrupt urinary function. Studies have demonstrated significant associations between constipation and lower urinary tract symptoms, thus illustrating the interrelationship between digestive and renal–urinary systems. See Al-hababi et al. (2021). *The Association Between Constipation and Lower Urinary Tract Symptoms in Parous Middle-Aged Women: A Prospective Cohort Study.*

181 *"Kidney function can block Heart function."* In chronic Kidney disease, impaired Kidney function reduces the body's ability to eliminate metabolic waste and regulate fluid and electrolyte balance. These disruptions then can lead to hypertension and volume overload, which in turn place significant strain on cardiac function and increase the risk of Heart failure. Recent studies have demonstrated a strong association between declining Kidney function and the development of Heart failure, particularly in older adults. See Buyadaa et al. (2025), *Kidney Function and Risk of Heart Failure in Older Adults: Findings from a Prospective Cohort Study.*

182 *"Overloaded Heart suppresses Lung function."* Respiratory distress is often among the earliest clinical signs of congestive Heart failure, reflecting the close physiological interdependence between cardiac and pulmonary systems. See Ahmad et al. (2024), *The Interplay of Heart Failure and Lung Disease: Clinical Correlations, Mechanisms, and Therapeutic Implications.*

Chapter 8: The Heart and Spine 心膂

The Heart

According to the *Liùjīng* 《六經》 (*Six Classics*),[183] the Chinese word for Heart, *xīn* 心, is a pictogram of the Heart organ, which corresponds to what is known as the "king of shapes" and "master of spirit."[184] As we saw in the previous chapter, the Heart is one of the five organ networks, along with Spleen, Lung, Kidney and Liver. According to the *Internal Medicine Classic*, "the nature of the Heart belongs to the Fire phase."[185] The relationships of the five phases represent the physiologic functioning of both generation (*shēng* 生) and control (*kè* 克) of the five organ networks, which can be proven by evidence and easily understood.[186] The use of the five phases to represent the interactivity between the five organs is a conceptual framework[187] which provides a system for explaining the principles of cause and effect. From this it can be seen that even five thousand years ago, East Asian medicine had developed a sophisticated set of natural scientific principles that should not be regarded lightly. East Asian medicine considers the relationship of the five internal organ networks in the same ways as it does the principles of generating and overcoming (*shēng* and *kè*) the five phases in Nature. This framework is based on the holistic ideas described in the *Yìjīng* 《易經》 *(Book of Changes)*:

"Heaven, Earth and Humanity are under one principle."[188]

It cannot be said in two or three words, but suffice it to say here that none of these relationships will be found to go beyond the boundaries of *yīn-yáng* and the five phases (*wǔ xíng* 五行). In Heaven, it is the movement of the sun, moon and five stars. On Earth, it is the behavior of animals, plants, mountains and streams. Among humans, it is man, woman and the five relationships.[189] Neither Heaven, Earth or Human depart from the dynamics of *yīn-yáng* and the five phases (*wǔ xíng*). The principle of generating and overcoming within the five organ-networks and their correspondence with the five phases must be studied in the *Internal Medicine Classic (Nèijīng)*. It cannot be explained here briefly.[190]

The Nature and Function of the Human Heart

According to a report by the US Department of Health, one person dies of Heart disease in Taiwan every two minutes.[191] The seriousness of the health of this organ is therefore obvious. I wish to briefly introduce here an analysis and physiological explanation of Heart disease as understood by Chinese medical experts in order to shed some light on the similarities and differences to Western medicine as a reference for patients and doctors alike. I hope that the contemporary medical world will take note of it and offer their own insights for the benefit of mankind.

The treatment of the human Heart in East Asian medicine is based upon the interrelationship of the five internal organs corresponding to that of the five phases. As discussed in the previous chapter, its objective is to understand Heart disease based on the principle of mutual generating and overcoming cycles found in Nature. Direct treatment (of the Heart) is considered secondary. When treating Heart disease, consideration is given to the interrelationship of all five organ networks to help them reach harmony and equilibrium, much like positioning of king and ministers of a nation in their respective places. Therefore, just targeting the Heart alone is never considered enough.

As explained earlier, the five phases correspond to the five organ networks, and the Heart is considered to belong to the Fire phase; the Liver corresponds to the Wood phase which can produce Fire, thus acting like mother to the Heart; the Spleen corresponds to the Earth phase, which acts as child of the Heart; the Kidney corresponds to the Water phase, which acts like the controller of the Heart; the Lung corresponds to the Metal phase, which is directly under the influence and control of the Heart. One must first examine the cause of an organ's loss of function, then find the evidence of its excess or deficiency and determine which phase is involved in its health and safety as well as its danger, and finally, decide upon the method of eliminating the excess and supplementing the deficiency. This is called "holistic healing."[192]

In cases where one's life force[193] is used up, the patient is not just given a prescription for medicine but is advised to seek the aid of a master. This is what *Huátuó* 華佗 (140–208 CE)[194] meant by his statement: "One can only treat disease but not save a life." Thus, in treating diseases, a doctor of East Asian medicine is expected to do only what is humanly possible. If doctors want to understand which organ networks are exerting the most influence on the Heart's dysfunction, they should first look at the Kidney and Liver, respectively. The other organ networks (Spleen and Lung) may be considered afterward.[195] Since everyone must eat and drink, what a patient eats and drinks corresponds to the five flavors (*wǔ wèi* 五味).[196] And since the five flavors correspond to the five organs and five phases, dietary interventions are first used to understand causes and augment the treatment.

The basic flavor associated with the Heart is bitterness.[197] Tea is bitter, liquor also contains bitterness, as do coffee and tobacco. Most men are extremely fond of these and unwilling to give them up. In particular, opium and morphine, which are extremely bitter and poisonous, are known by everyone to be harmful to the human body and yet some people are willing to risk their lives to indulge in them. This is because physiologically, the Heart is so attracted to the taste of bitterness and therefore the desire easily becomes habit.[198] Not only is the Heart associated with a specific flavor that it resonates with, but the other four organs do as well. Each is associated with an altogether different flavor. The Spleen is fond of sweetness, the Lungs are fond of savory (aromatic) spices, the Kidneys are fond of saltiness and the Liver is fond of sour or tart flavors. These are the basic five flavors that correspond to the five organ networks. If a man loves his food salty, his Kidneys must be particularly strong. But if the Kidneys become too strong, the corresponding Water phase has a tendency of putting out the Fire, thus excess salt can injure the Heart. If a person loves sour food, his Liver is particularly strong, and the corresponding Wood phase has the tendency to generate Fire thus benefitting the Heart. This is called the benefits and losses (to an organ) according to the five phase principle of generating and controlling. The cumulative effects of diet do not happen in one day. It takes a person decades or even a whole lifetime of habits to manifest these imbalances. Since the causes of disease can sometimes take a long time to develop, the longer it's present, the harder it is to cure. So those who wish to strengthen their Hearts must pay close attention to their daily habits in order to reap later benefits.

For instance, the Liver is said to be like the mother of the Heart. How does a person protect the Liver, which corresponds to the Wood phase? I believe that besides making good use of sour flavors in one's food and drink, one must also seek relaxation and a broad outlook.[199] Worry and narrow-mindedness are inappropriate. Because the sinews and tendons are affected by the Liver, the Heart [and circulatory system] should be like the branches of a tree, which stretch out loosely and comfortably. One must therefore avoid tension which tightens the muscles, tendons and blood vessels thus raising blood pressure. It is especially important to think about forgiveness as well. If one can add some light and limbering exercises, doing some loosening of the tendons and activating the muscles, as *Zhuāngzǐ* said of "the bear hanging and bird stretching," while maintaining open-hearted self-awareness, this will allow the *qì* and blood to flow naturally. This would be most beneficial to the Heart.[200]

Furthermore, in seeking peace of mind, self-cultivation should be guided by these four words:

率性任真
"Draw out one's original nature to be true."[201]

As stated before, the nature of the Heart is Fire, and Fire represents bright and clear light. It is like the sun shining in the sky. Even the slightest cloud or fog obscures its light. That is why the *Book of History*[202] says:

立作偽則心勞日拙
"If you start out being false (to yourself),[203]
your Heart/mind will become increasingly dull day by day."

These words reveal the key to many psychological disorders.[204] When one's life is contrived, one cannot escape from sacrificing one's integrity and injuring one's original nature, much like the sun being obscured by an overcast sky. This results in the destruction of one's mental and psychological well being. How then can one ever achieve peace of mind? Furthermore, if one truly desires peace of mind, one cannot do better than sinking the Heart/mind into the *dāntián* 丹田 and letting the breath settle there; keeping calm and remaining quiet.

If one's Heart/mind function is unbalanced or is attacked directly by other conditions, the causes must be carefully examined, ascertained, and then a remedy decided upon. Only then, after doing everything humanly possible to remedy the situation, if the Heart's *qì* remains exhausted, then it's time to stop treatment.

If another person's Heart is used to replace (transplant) it in order to temporarily prolong life, it is possible to revitalize the Heart organ by the application of extraordinary medical skill but if the other four organ networks are already in deteriorated condition, the restoration of health will be short-lived and the application of the most wonderful surgical skill will be of no real help. I have always regarded the early death of Yan Hui[205] and the short life of *Kǒng Míng* 孔明[206] as matters of regret, for they were not able to complete their usefulness. But, even if their Hearts could have been replaced and their lives extended, I must say that they would no longer be Yán Huí and Kǒng Míng. So what is to be valued and what is to be regretted? The most valued thing in a human life is his spirit-intelligence (*líng* 靈).[207] Once it is used up, it matters not whether he lives or dies. Like grain, when it ripens early, there is an early harvest; when it ripens late, there is a late harvest. After the grain is harvested, the rest is all just stalks and roots, which may be discarded. Therefore, the best to be expected from a good physician is to help one live out one's natural life and be contented with that. I am wondering how these words of mine will be understood by learned people![208]

Equal Emphasis on Heart and Spine[209]

The *Internal Medicine Classic* treats the vessels *Rèn* 任 and *Dū* 督 with equal emphasis.[210] The *Shūjīng* 《書經》 *(Book of History)* also mentions Heart and spine together.[211] Daoist practices go into great detail concerning the relationship of one's Heart/mind and spine (*Rèn* and *Dū)* in self-cultivation. *Tàijí quán* is an internal form of exercise. It was said to have been developed by the Daoist sage *Zhāng Sānfēng* 張三丰 ([212] in the late Song Dynasty by following Lǎozǐ and Emperor Huang's principle of "creating action through non-action"[213] in combination with the *Book of Changes'* principle of *lǐ, qì, xiàng* 理氣象.[214] Its fundamental meaning directly pertains to the *Rèn* and *Dū* vessels which govern the "eight extraordinary vessels" (*qíjīng bāmài* 奇經八脈)[215] (see Figure 22).

The *Rèn* vessel is linked to the Heart and governs the functions of one's mind whereas the *Dū* vessel is linked to the Kidneys and governs the bodily form.[216] In essence, the connection between these two vessels reveals how form and function are united; the spine (and Kidneys, marrow, brain) relating to form; the Heart/mind relating to function. When considered as a whole, this is the entire focus of *tàijí quán* practice. It is for this reason, that *tàijí quán* is considered a superior form of exercise.

Thus the Heart/mind serves as master of the physical form.[217] The teachings of the sages emphasize, *"letting your Heart relax."*[218] Zen Buddhists always ask, *"Is the master home?"* By "master" is meant the Heart/mind. These teachings are more or less similar to what the Daoists refer to as the union of Heart and Kidney networks.[219] Stated in different ways respectively, they all carry the same meaning. But *tàijí quán* goes one step further. That is, this principle is actually and clearly demonstrated through movement. The reason I add this chapter on the equal emphasis on Heart/mind and spine is to illustrate the fact that function does not exist without form.

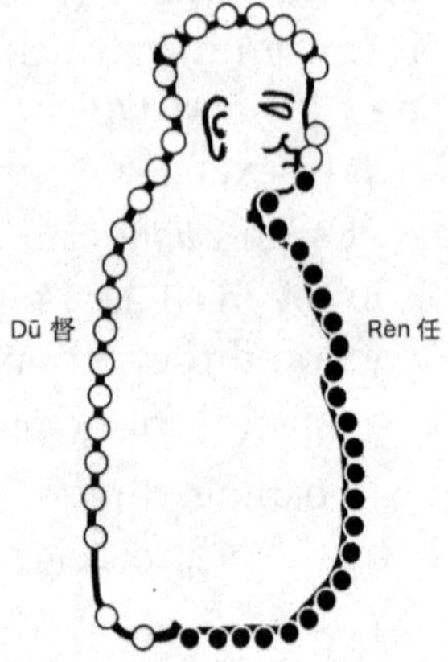

Figure 22 Illustration of Rèn and Dū Vessels
by Ed Young (white dots are *yáng*, black dots are *yīn*)

When we speak of " Heart," we do not mean simply the organ Heart, but the Heart/mind-spirit.[220] The two are not separate entities and yet they are not one and the same, either. That the organ-Heart can function and give spirit to other organs depends on the Heart/mind-spirit.

The Spinal Column in Relation to the Heart

Now as for the spine,[221] it has twenty-four vertebrae and forms the main skeletal column with numerous sections. Not only are the five organs and the six viscera connected with it,[222] but it also serves as the main support for the five limbs of the body.[223] For self-cultivation and health, the spine must be given major consideration. It is also a fundamental concern in *tàijí quán*. The beginner should practice having Heart/mind (spirit) and *qì* (breath) guard each other within the *dāntián* without using force or losing focus. This is what is meant by "letting the Heart relax" and "the master is at home."

After practicing this for a long time, the *jīngqì* 精氣 will be able to pass through the sacrum, penetrate the spine, move up and pass through the base of the skull[224] to reach the top of the brain. From there it returns down the front of the body back to the *dāntián*. This is what is meant by communication of *Rèn* and *Dū* and union of Heart-spirit and Kidney.[225] But this state cannot be reached in one day or one night. It must occur naturally and never be forced. If this is accomplished, not only can the practice of *tàijí quán* reach the highest degree of attainment, preventing sickness and prolonging life, but one's spirit can be preserved without deterioration.

Although it is difficult to speak about the Heart/mind, many scholars and practitioners of self-cultivation have explained what was spoken of by former sages as "educating the Heart" and "centering the Heart" and "not affecting the Heart," which are as clear as the sun and moon appearing in the sky and which can be learned easily without detailing it here.[226] Generally speaking the ancients said:

"In meditative self-cultivation, one must sit erect properly and maintain one's demeanor"[227]

Many explanations have been given for the meaning of "sitting erect" during meditation and yet not one has mentioned the element of risk of injury. But I think there surely is an element of danger here. The spine consists of many bones strung like a string of beads resting one on top of another. If one is not careful, leaning will cause it to become crooked and protruding.[228] Then it will lose its strength and not be able to support the structural branches of one's body. This may result in an assortment of diseases, such as herniations and in extreme cases will result in collapse like the "falling of the main pillar of a house." Is this not an element of danger? Those experienced in practicing meditation know of this danger. They try to avoid the slightest leaning in order to prevent such injuries. We have a saying that one must walk "as if on the edge of a precipice," or "as if walking on thin ice." "To sit erect in a dignified manner"[229] implies maintaining an erect spine to avoid sickness. Being wary of danger will prevent falling, which could cause further injury. I believe that improper sitting indeed poses real dangers, since a tense spine that has many joints can lead to unfavorable postures, often resulting in severe discomfort or awkward gait. When one has lost the natural curvature of the spine, it can lead to problems supporting and balancing the body. Hence, if the spine gradually diminishes into a state of weakness, it can truly cause illness. To avoid such problems, one should maintain a proper posture while sitting. In *tàijí* I always say, the spine should be upright; if one is leaning sideways, it is just like being tight and overbearing. All illnesses manifest this way; understanding the danger can help mitigate it.

Note: Ed and I came upon this rhymed poem, scrawled on a scrap of paper among Professor Cheng notes. It turns out to be a well-known rhyming proverb about meditation.

lì rú sōng
立如松
Stand like a pine

zuò rú zhōng
坐如鐘
Sit like a bell

wò rú gōng
臥如弓
Sleep like a bow

xíng rú fēng
行如風
Walk like the wind[230]

Ch. 8 Notes

---

183 The *Liùjīng* 《六經》(*Six Classics*) consist of the, *Yìjīng* 《易經》(*Book of Changes*), *Shàngshū* 《尚書》(*Book of History*), *Lǐjì* 《禮記》(*Book of Rites*), *Book of Songs* (*Shījīng* 《詩經》), *the Chūnqiū zuǒzhuàn* 《春秋左傳》(*Spring and Autumn Annals*). The fifth *Lèjì* 《樂記》(*Book of Music*) is now lost.

---

184 "Spirit" here is *shén* 神 (see Chapters 4 & 5). When the Heart (*xīn* 心) is understood as the anatomic organ of circulation, *shén* expresses itself as a sense of flowing vitality. When Heart is defined as "mind" this *Shén* gives a sense of consciousness, imagination, and the ability to extend one's thoughts beyond the material world. As Peter Firebrace describes: "*The Heart as pivot between the spiritual and mental faculties, calm seat of the emotions. Empty, to receive, unobstructed, to allow the free flow of life on every level*" Larre and Rochat de La Valee (1991), *The Heart*, p. ii. See Appendix III: *Etymological Glossary of Sage Principle Terms* for descriptions of the characters *xīn* 心 (Heart-mind) and *shén* 神 (spirit).

185 "The Heart belongs to the Fire phase" According to the system of correspondence as stated in chapter five of the *Huáng Dì Nèijīng Sùwèn* 《黃帝內經素問》 "*In the Heavens [the Heart] constitutes heat. On Earth, it engenders Fire, among the physical constituents, the vessels, among the zang organs, the Heart*" Wilms (2018), *Humming with Elephants: The Great Treatise on the Resonant Manifestations of Yin and Yang*, p. 176.

186 See *shēng* and *kè* cycles in Chapter 7.

187 The conceptual framework referred to here is the organization of relationships referred to in the five phase diagram (see Chapter 7) with its underlying logic and functional dynamics elaborated in Chapter 8.

188 This is Professor Cheng's summation of the quote from *Yìjīng* 《易經》 chapter "Discussing the Hexagrams" (*Shuo Guà Zhuan* 說卦傳 2), which states: "*In ancient times, the sages made the Book of Changes to follow the order of their nature and fate. Therefore they determined the Dao of the Heavens and named it yīn-yáng, determined the Dao of Earth and named it hardness and softness and determined the Dao of (Hu)man and named it benevolence and upright. They combined these three fundamental powers and doubled them, hence the Book of Changes hexagram (guà) is always formed by six lines.*" Adapted from Wilhelm (1987). *The I Ching or Book of Changes*, p. 264.

189 "The Five Relationships:" According to Confucian thought, each person has a specific place in society and certain duties to fulfill. These are described as the five principal relationships: (1) ruler and subject; (2) father and son; (3) elder brother and younger brother; (4) husband and wife; and (5) friend and friend. See Ames & Hall (2001). *Focusing the Familiar*, p. 38.

190 Throughout the *Huáng Dì Nèijīng Sùwèn* 《黃帝內經素問》 and in particular Chapter 5, it describes a holistic "systematic correspondence" of functions that exist in the macrocosm of seasonal weather conditions (heaven), in the same way as it does in the microcosm of human physical, emotional, cognitive and spiritual functions.

---

191 According to the Centers for Disease Control and Prevention (CDC), in 2012 approximately 600,000 people died from Heart disease in the United States each year, about one in every four deaths, or roughly one death every minute. This rate represents a significant increase from the estimates available to Professor Cheng when he was writing in the 1960s. More recent data show an even greater impact. In 2023, 919,032 people in the United States died from cardiovascular disease, accounting for approximately one in every three deaths. These figures are drawn from the National Center for Health Statistics (2025). *Multiple Cause of Death, 2018–2023 on the CDC WONDER Database.*

192 "Holistic healing" (*Quánti dàzhì* 全體大治). Literally "whole-body-great-healing" emphasizing a treatment approach that addresses the entire body and its interconnected systems rather than isolated symptoms.

193 "Life force" (*mìnggēn* 命根). Literally: "destiny-root" or "basis of life," refers to the vital essence or core of one's being, often understood as the things one cherishes and protects most in life.

194 *Huátuó* 華佗 (Huato; 140–208 CE), the legendary Han Dynasty physician traditionally credited with inventing anesthesia for surgery. He is also said to have developed the "Five Animal Frolics" (*wǔqínxì* 五禽戲), *qìgōng* 氣功 exercises that are believed to have health benefits. Recent research has confirmed the benefits of *qìgōng* in the treatment of chronic diseases. See Guo, Zhao, & Zhang (2018). *Beneficial Effects of Qigong Wuqinxi in the Improvement of Chronic Low Back Pain, Physical Fitness, and Quality of Life in the Elderly.*

195 If one refers to the five phase (*wǔxíng* 五行) diagram in the previous chapter, Kidney and Liver have direct influences on the Heart. Therefore, Professor Cheng recommends starting with these two relationships in managing Heart conditions.

196 Five flavors (*wǔ wèi* 五味) described in the system of correspondences according to the *Nèijīng* as salty, sour, bitter, sweet, savory aromatic corresponding to Water, Wood, Fire, Earth, and Metal, respectively.

197 "Bitterness" (*kǔ* 苦) meaning bitter flavor and also meaning hardship or suffering. Professor Cheng has presented the so called "three fearlessnesses," the first, to be "without fear of eating (taking on) bitterness" (*wúwei chī kǔ* 無畏喫苦). The image of *kǔ* is said to be a mouth consuming bitter herbs.

198 Chapter 5 of the *Nèijīng Sùwèn* states that "Fire engenders bitterness. Bitterness engenders the Heart…among the wills (desires) it is Happiness." 火生苦，苦生心…在志為喜 from Wilms (2018). *Humming with Elephants: The Great Treatise on the Resonant Manifestations of Yin and Yang,* p. 176. (Note: The Heart's endless desire for happiness has great bearing today on the opioid epidemic.)

---

199 Professor Cheng here is referencing the logic sequence of correspondences in *Huáng Dì Nèijīng Sùwèn* 《黃帝內經素問》 Chapter 5 *"Wood engenders sourness. Sourness engenders the Liver. The Liver engenders the sinews. The sinews engender the Heart. the Liver rules the eyes."* (東方生風，風生木，木生酸，酸生肝，肝生筋，筋生心，肝主目). ibid, p. 162.

200 *Bear-hanging and bird-stretching* in *Zhuāngzǐ* 莊子 refers to one of the foundational Daoists texts (5th-3rd BCE) Chapter 15 ("Constrained in Will") *"To repair to the thickets and ponds, living idly in the wilderness, angling for fish in solitary places, inaction (wuwei) his only concern - such is the life favored by the scholar of the rivers and seas, the man who withdraws from the world, the unhurried idler. To pant, to puff, to hail, to sip, to spit out the old breath and draw in the new, practicing bear-hangings and bird-stretchings, longevity his only concern - such is the life favored by the scholar who practices "induction," the man who nourishes his body, who hopes to live to be as old as Pengzu* 所好" see Watson, (1968). *The Complete Works of Chuang Tzu*, p. 167. (就藪澤，處閒曠，釣魚閒處，無為而已矣，此江海之士，避世之人，閒暇者之所好也。吹呴呼吸，吐故納新，熊經鳥申，為壽而已矣，此道引之士，養形之人，彭祖壽考者之所好也.)

Note: It is thought that these breathing techniques and body exercises relate to early *dǎoyǐn* 导引exercises that form the basis of *tàijí* 太極, and *qìgōng* 氣功 practices). For more on the medical benefits of *qìgōng* related to the health of the Heart, blood circulation and spine, see Chen, et al. (2019). *Dao Yin (a.k.a. Qigong): Origin, development, potential mechanisms, and clinical applications.*

201 *Shuai Xìng Rèn Zhēn* 率 性 任 真 literal translation: "lead/draw out one's original nature to bear truth." This appears to be Professor's distillation of the opening quote from the Confucian Doctrine of the Mean (Zhōngyōng 中庸) which itself is considered to have been derived from "an oft-cited apothegm that…belongs to a collection of pre-Mencian textual materials associated with the name of Confucius's grandson, Zisi: *"What Heaven (tian) commands (ming) is called "natural tendencies" (xing); drawing out these natural tendencies is called the proper way (dao); improving upon this way is called education"* (天命之謂性，率性之謂道) Ames & Hall (2001). *Focusing the Familiar a Translation and Philosophical Interpretation of the Zhongyong*, p. 26. See Appendix III: *Etymological Glossary of Sage Principle Terms*, for a more detailed analysis of *Xìng* 性 *Rèn* 任 *Zhēn* 真.

202 The *Shūjīng* 《書經》 *(Classic of History)*: also known as the *Shàngshū* 《尚書》 from the Spring and Autumn period (772-476 BCE) is one of the five classics of ancient Chinese literature. The exact source for this phrase is unclear. It appears to be Professor Cheng's own take on a quote from Chapter 3 of the *Hànshū* 《漢書》 *(The Book of Han).*

---

203 *Wèi* 偽: Literally, "man-made," often translated as "false," "artificial," "forged," "fake," or "contrived." Professor Cheng draws an intriguing contrast between true and false (*zhēn* 真 and *wèi* 偽), particularly as these concepts relate to the authenticity of one's original nature (*xìng* 性).

204 Emphasis here is on the unique East Asian mind-body perspective of Heart (*xin* 心) as an organ of both soma and psyche.

205 Yán Huí 顏回 (521-481 BCE) was a devoted student of Confucius. According to tradition, by the age of twenty-nine, his hair had already turned completely white, and he died prematurely at thirty-two. He is venerated as one of the Four Sages of Confucianism (*sì pèi* 四配), which include Yán Huí 顏回(521-481 BCE), Zēngzǐ 曾子 (personal name Zēng Shēn 曾參; 505-435 BCE), Zǐsī 子思 (personal name Kǒng Jí 孔伋; 481-402 BCE), Mèngzǐ 孟子 (personal name Mèng Kē 孟軻; 372-289 BCE).

206 Kǒng Míng 孔明 (K'ung-ming), also known as Zhūgě Liàng 諸葛亮 (181-234 CE), was a renowned sage and strategist of the Three Kingdoms period (220–280 CE). He was a favorite figure of Professor Cheng, who often employed his oracle book for divination and forecasting.

207 *Líng* 靈: "spirited," "cleverness," "alertness," or "intelligence." (See Chapter 4 and Appendix III: *Etymological Glossary of Sage Principle Terms*, for a more detailed analysis of these characters.)

208 Professor Cheng was writing during the 1960s at a time when Western medicine was making great advances in keeping the body alive with such things as heart transplants, and he is pondering the merit of such procedures.

209 "Spine" (lǚ 膂) the term Professor Cheng is using here is similar to the character *dū* 督: the channel that runs along the spine. Professor Cheng is emphasizing the equal importance of spinal cord and the Heart from the perspective of the front midline and back midline in maintaining health and balance of the mind/body. (See Footnote 24 *Rèn* and *Dū*.)

210 *Rèn* 任, in East Asian medicine this is referred to as the "conception vessel," or "controller" (Unschuld) which runs along the front midline of the body. *Rèn* ideogram is said to depict a person carrying a weighted pole, which can also represent the unity of Heaven-Earth-Humanity. *Rèn* means "to bear, duty, trust to, rely on." It is considered *yīn* relative to the *yáng* of the *Dū* spinal vessel. *Dū* 督 in East Asian medicine often translated as the "governing vessel" or "supervisor" (Unschuld) travels up the spine. *Dū* ideogram depicts a hand picking beans above the image of an eye, conveying the meaning "to oversee," "supervise," "superintend," or "govern." *Dū* and *Rèn* vessels are part of the eight Extraordinary Vessels that make up the so called "microcosmic orbit" discussed later in this book. See Appendix III: *Etymological Glossary of Sage Principle Terms*, for a more detailed analysis of the ideogram of *Rèn* & *Dū*.

---

211 *Shūjīng* 《書經》 *(Book of History)* writes: *"The trembling anxiety of my mind makes me feel as if I were treading on a tiger's tail, or walking upon spring ice. I now give you charge to assist me; be as my limbs to me, as my Heart and backbone"* (心之憂危，若蹈虎尾，涉于春冰。今命爾予翼，作股肱心膂). From Chapter 1 in *Zhōu Shū* 周書 - Section: *Jūn Yá* 君牙, Legge (1879). *The Sacred Books of the East vol. III*, pp. 250-251.

212 *Zhāng Sānfēng* 張三丰 legendary Daoist sage who is said to have observed a hawk/crane attacking a snake and was greatly inspired by the snake's defensive tactics. See Davis (2004). *The Taiji quan Classics: An Annotated Translation*, p. 17.

213*"Creating action through inaction"* (*wúwéi ránhòu yǒu wéi* 無為然後有為) is similar to *wéi wúwéi* 為無為 literally: "doing without doing," the Daoist doctrine of allowing things to take their own natural course without meddling, "doing that is free of coercive manipulation." Ames & Hall (2003), *Dao De Jing: A Philosophical Translation*. This quote is found in both *Lǎozǐ* and *Zhuāngzǐ* texts.

214 See Chapter 3: Lǐ, Qì, Xiàng 理氣象.

215 Eight Extraordinary Vessels (*qíjīng bāmài* 奇經八脈) are often considered a subsystem of the East Asian medicine meridian system that act as reservoirs thought to derive from Daoist cultivation practices.

216 See five phase correspondence of Kidney/adrenal/urogenital to Water in previous chapter, Chapter 7.

217 *"The Heart/mind serves as master of the physical form."* In classical Chinese medicine, the relation of *Rèn* and *Dū* vessels corresponds to the relationship of Heart and Kidney, considered a relative *yīn-yáng* (front/back) relationship, each being master over the other. Heart and Kidney have a relative correspondence between "mind" and "brain" that also relates to the fundamental relationship of Fire and Water discussed in the final *Yìjīng* 《易經》 Hexagrams 63 ䷾ and 64 ䷿.

218 *"letting your Heart relax" fàngxīn* 放心 "to feel relieved; to feel reassured; to be at ease," *fàng* 放 - "to let go, to release, to free, to liberate, to loosen, to relax." Lǎozǐ Ch. 3 also emphasizes a form of relaxing the Heart/mind (*xūxīn* 虛心), "emptying one's Heart/mind." *Xūxīn* carries an implied sense of humility important to both Daoists and Confucianists. *Huáng Dì Nèijīng Sùwèn* 《黃帝內經素問》 Chapter 17 mentions emptying the mind in the context of open-minded sensing *"to feel [the movement in] the vessels has a Way: emptiness (open-mindedness) and quietude are to be treasured."* (Unschuld & Tessenow (2011), *Huang Di Nei Jing Su Wen: An Annotated Translation of Huang Di's Inner Classic*, p. 287.) In Zen practice this relaxed and clear-mindedness is referred to as "empty mind" *kōngxīn* 空心 (See *Heart Sūtra* [*Xīnjīng* 《心經》] verse).

---

219 *The union of Heart and Kidney.* In East Asian medicine the Heart and Kidney form an intimate union known as the "Lesser Yin" (*shǎoyīn* 少陰), a component of the differentiation of the channels according to the "Six Conformations" or "Six Levels" formulated by Zhāng Zhòngjǐng 張仲景 in his *Shānghán Lùn* 傷寒論 (*Treatise on Cold Damage*).

220 "Heart/mind-spirit (*xīnlíng* 心靈) literally "bright; smart; quick-witted; Heart; thoughts; spirit," this carries the idea of mind/body unity.

221 "Spine" (*jǐ* 脊): Here Professor Cheng is differentiating the spinal column from the spinal cord, that is, the boney structure from the *Dū* channel proper. See Appendix III: *Etymological Glossary of Sage Principle Terms*, for a more detailed analysis of these characters.

222 From a Western anatomical perspective, the spinal column contains the nerves that innervate the internal organs via the sympathetic and parasympathetic nerve bundles that emerge from it.

223 "The five limbs" are the head and four extremities.

224 The "Jade pillow" (*yùzhěn* 玉枕) is located at the base of the skull (see transformation of *jīng* 精 Chapter 5 and Chapter 13).

225 Note in East Asian medicine the Kidney-Heart makes up the central energetic axis that corresponds to *jīngshén* 精神, the primal orientation of essence and spirit. Genetic heredity and consciousness are a microcosm of Earth-Heaven, and *yīn-yáng*, respectively. In East Asian medicine add *qì* 氣 as the interface between the *jīng* 精 and *shén* 神; to make *jīng-qì-shén*, the so-called "three treasures" (*sānbǎo* 三寶,) that is a reflection of the functional unity of Earth-Human-Heaven trinity, respectively.

226 Ed Young's note: "Educating the Heart," "centering the Heart," and "not affecting the Heart" are Confucian, Daoist and Zen terms for cultivation practices that refer to emptying biases and prejudices and not exercising one's will over circumstances or using force. This is literally translated as "correcting the Heart" (*zhèngxīn* 正心), " Heart transmission" (*xīnchuán jí* 心傳及) "Heart unmoved by anything" (*měi bù dòngxīn* 每不動心), respectively. The Heart/mind in East Asian medicine is considered an empty vessel. This allows for free-flowing circulatory function. When we push too hard, we end up with excessive symptoms of physical strain (high blood pressure, headache etc.) and emotional stress (anxiety, distress, depression etc.) and distorted/biased thinking."

227 "To sit erect" refers to sitting meditation practices; this is just sitting quietly and observing as a matter of cultivation. For information on this see Neo-Confucian philosopher Yáng Shí 楊時 (1053–1135) in Song (2024), *Yang Shi's Confucian quiet-sitting meditation: A Distinction from Cheng Yi and Huayan Buddhism.*

---

[228] *Qū tū* 曲凸: Literally "crooked and protruding." These were favorite characters of Ed's in his teaching of *tàijí*. See Appendix III: *Etymological Glossary of Sage Principle Terms*, for a more detailed analysis of these characters.

[229] Literally "with straightened gown."

[230] Daniel Schrier, editor: From a Daoist perspective, these "Four Postures" (*sìzhǒng zīshì* 四種姿勢) cultivate alignment, sacred connection, and energetic integration, ensuring the smooth circulation of qi throughout the body during *yǎngshēng* 養生 ("nourishing life") or meditation practice. "Walk like the wind." You cannot show what wind looks like. You only perceive it through its effects, how it moves leaves, bends grasses, passes through valleys. Wind itself is invisible. We see this in *fēng shuǐ* 風水 ("wind and water") which describes the movement of qi through a landscape. The same is true of the body: we do not see qi directly, we experience how it moves. To walk like the wind is to move without obstruction. Wind flows in all directions. It does not resist; it adapts. It passes through openings, wraps around obstacles, and continues on its way. When walking embodies this quality, movement becomes responsive rather than forced, light, adaptive, and alive. Thus, "to walk like the wind" is not merely a physical instruction. It is an energetic one. When the body is relaxed, qi moves freely. When qi moves freely, the body becomes like the wind, ungraspable, unobstructed, and quietly powerful.

The Daoist principle for standing refers not to trees in general (*shù* 樹) but specifically to the pine tree (*sōng* 松). This evokes the character *sōng* 鬆, meaning "relaxation," composed of *biāo* 彡 ("unbound long hair") above *sōng* 松 ("pine"), with the latter typically read as a phonetic. What is the body like when it is truly relaxed? Rooted yet open, stable yet flexible, and able to receive movement rather than resist it. Beyond its linguistic nuance, the evergreen pine tree symbolizes longevity and even immortality in Daoism. To "stand like a pine" is to cultivate rootedness, extension, and suppleness simultaneously.

To "sit like a bell" is to embody stability and quiet strength. The bell being invoked is large, grounded, and hollow at its center. When placed on the earth, it rests firmly, unmoving, solid and strong on the outside, yet open and empty within. This image guides how we sit: the body rooted and supported, the structure stable, while the inside remains spacious and relaxed. The outer form (bones, posture, and alignment) provides strength; the inner body (muscles, flesh, breath) stays soft and responsive, connected to the earth. To "sit like a bell" is to balance firmness with emptiness, and "grounded-ness" with ease.

In Daoist practice, "to sleep like a bow" describes a particular sleeping position. Typically lying on the right side, the right leg extended, the left leg slightly bent. The right hand supports the head under the ear, while the left hand rests gently between the thighs.The curvature of the body mirrors the bow's form, arched, protected, yet flexible. This shape is not only protective, like a turtle shell, but also functional. It supports the return of the Hun, the ethereal soul, to the Liver. It encourages the Liver's restorative work, purifying the blood, smoothing the flow of qi, and facilitating dream consciousness.

Chapter 9: The Dāntián 丹田[231]

Forty years ago, when I wrote the book entitled *Thirteen Chapters on Tai Chi Quan*,[232] I was told by a friend, Mr. Tsao Soong 曹松,[233] that a French physician who practiced surgery for twenty years had found the location of what Daoists called the *dāntián*. There is a membrane, which forms a pocket-like sac between the large and small intestines. Among athletes and fighters, this membrane is thicker and the sac is enlarged to the size of a man's fist. At that time, I used these findings as physiological proof of what had been discussed in China for centuries as *dāntián* and included it in my book. Since then more medical information has become available to me for better understanding.

Dāntián is a technical name used by Daoists. Lǎozǐ has explained it quite clearly in the *Huángtíng jīng* 《黃庭經》 *(Classic of the Yellow Court)*.[234] In the *Huáng Dì Nèijīng* 《黃帝內經》 *(Yellow Emperor's Internal Medicine Classic)*, it is called by the name "Sea of Qì."[235] Western medicine calls it the "omentum[236] (see Figure 23). It has been noted that this omentum forms a sac that moves to protect the different parts of the abdomen from threatening influences.[237] For instance, during operations on the abdominal region, this membrane will shift to cover the area of incision in order to protect the area. In cases of appendicitis, this membranous sac covers the diseased organ and helps to wall it off and protect the rest of the body.[238]

The illustrations that follow (Figures 23 & 24) are based on the standard medical text, *Cunningham's Textbook of Anatomy*

(1964). In Figure 24, the dotted lines indicate the prenatal development of this sac. The movement of the omentum, in response to pressures or forces external to it, matches my original explanation.

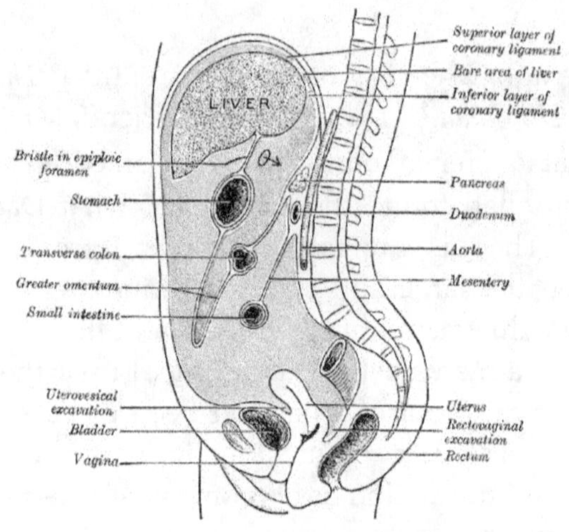

Figure 23: Omentum (side view)
(from Cunningham's Textbook of Anatomy, 1964)

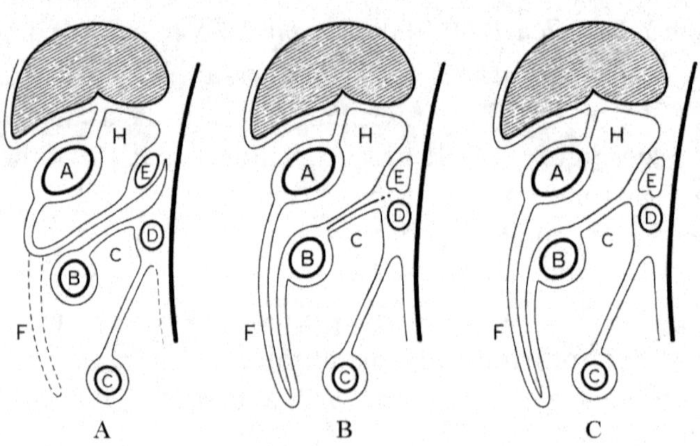

Figure 24: Embryologic Development of Omentum
(adapted from Cunningham's Textbook of Anatomy, 1964)

The cross-section diagram of the abdomen (left side is the front, right side is the back) based on *Cunningham's Textbook of Anatomy* shows the *dāntián* (F) also known as the "sea of qì" which corresponds to the omentum in Western medical nomenclature. Figure A shows the lesser omentum (H) with the embryologic beginning of the greater omentum (F-dotted line extending down from the Stomach, and Figure B shows the developing omentum (F) extending down from Stomach (A); in front of the transverse colon (B); and small intestine (C); duodenum (D); and the pancreas (E). In Figure C the fully grown greater omentum (F) protects the peritoneal cavity. The potential space within the omental bursa (Sea of Qì) connects above with the lesser omentum, the so-called "Yellow Court" space (H) (*huángtíng* 黄庭*)* behind the Stomach (A).

From its location and its behavior, I have concluded that the omentum is what the Chinese *Internal Medicine Classic Neijing* calls the "Sea of Qì," and the Daoists call the *dāntián*. The reason that it can move involuntarily to resist threatening external and internal forces is the action of *qì*. Since there is no recognition of *qì* in the English-speaking world, this diagram merely proves the existence of the *dāntián*. However, to study the activity of the omentum and its principles requires further explanation below.

Dāntián 丹田 and *Huángtíng* 黄庭

According to the physiology described by Western medical sciences, there are two areas within the human internal organs that are considered inactive. One is a sac-like membrane within the abdomen, called the "Greater Omentum."[239] The other is an area, yellowish in color, that extends from the lower back near the left Kidney and extends up between the Spleen and pancreas to the Liver and diaphragm called the "Lesser Omentum."[240] It too is considered inactive.[241]

However, in East Asian medicine and Daoism, these two areas (though appearing inactive) are considered to play crucial roles in the human body.

The greater omentum is called the *dāntián* and the lesser omentum is called the "Yellow Court" (*huángtíng*).[242] The names are given differently by Chinese and Western medicine, but their location, shape and color indicate that they undoubtedly designate the same parts. I wish to explain a little of their functions.

East Asian medicine emphasizes the functioning of *qì* transformation. Since the West has not paid attention to this, it cannot easily comprehend its function. The *Huáng Dì Nèijīng* 《黃帝內經》*(Yellow Emperor's Internal Medicine Classic)* was said to be composed at the time of the Yellow Emperor (*Huáng Dì* 黃帝), five thousand years ago.[243] During the Warring states period,[244] *Lǎozǐ* 老子 followed Emperor Huáng's teachings to develop the *Dàodé jīng* 《道德經》 and later Daoists composed the *Huángtíng jīng* 《黃庭經》 *(Classic of the Yellow Court)*. Both books spoke of the wonderful functioning of the *dāntián* and *huángtíng*, which involve the principle of *yīn-yáng* dynamics as well as the five phases. One cannot understand East Asian physiology without comprehending these principles. They concern the fundamentals of life and require concentrated practice to be understood. For our present purpose it suffices to point out that East Asian and Western medicine may have different names for the same parts of human anatomy and yet their understanding of their respective functions is very different.

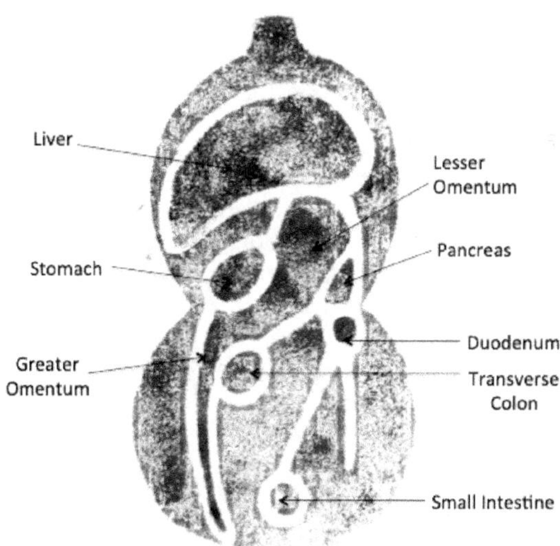

Figure 25: The Dāntián Within a Cross-section of the Abdomen with Anatomic Landmarks of the Omentum
Ed Young's artistic interpretation based on Professor Cheng's description

Ch. 9 Notes

---

231 *Dāntián* 丹田: lit. the cinnabar/elixir field - this represents the source of Daoist alchemy. It's access point is said to be located just below and behind the umbilicus. See Appendix III: *Etymological Glossary of Sage Principle Terms,* for a more detailed analysis of these characters.

232 See Cheng, Lo, & Inn. (1985). *Cheng Tzu's Thirteen Chapters on T'ai-chi Ch'uan.*

---

233 Tsao Soong 曹松 - In *Thirteen Chapters on Tai Chi Quan* (1982), Chapter 2, Tsao Soong was referred to as Cáo Zhòngshì 曹仲氏 by Professor Cheng.

234 The *Huángtíng jīng* 《黃庭經》 (*Huang T'ing Ching; Classic of the Yellow Court*) is a well-known Daoist text on meditation and internal alchemy. In the very first chapter of *Huáng Dì Nèijīng Sùwèn* 《黃帝內經素問》 *(Yellow Emperor's Internal Medicine Classic)* entitled "Discourse on the True Qì [Endowed by] Heaven" (上古天真論), reference is made to "True Qì" (*tiānzhēn* 天真). Paul Unschuld notes: "*The Daoists, in the Huang Ting Jing (*黃庭經*), have a saying: 'When the essence is concentrated and the qì is accumulated, this is the true [state]'"(*積精累氣以為真*). The notion expressed here is that of essence and qì being initially unseparated. Now True Qì (*天真*) refers to the essence-qì acquired prior to one's birth; it is the primordial matter underlying the vital activities of the human body*" Unschuld and Tessenow (2011), p. 29.

The oldest copy of the *Huángtíng jīng* is said to have been made by Wáng Xīzhī 王羲之, (303–379), though legend attributes its authorship to the Daoist mystic Lady Wèi Huácún 魏華存 (Wei Hua-Ts'un). According to myth, Lady Wei became interested in the teachings of Lǎozǐ 老子 and Zhuāngzǐ 莊子 at a young age and was instructed in the Daoist practice of *Huángtíng* 黃庭 (Yellow Court) meditation. This meditation emphasizes fortifying the Spleen, referred to as the "Yellow Court" because yellow is the color associated with the Earth elemental phase, which corresponds to the Spleen in East Asian cosmology. Strengthening the Spleen through this practice is believed to promote health and longevity. The *Huángtíng jīng* is also mentioned in Richard Wilhelm's translation of the *Secret of the Golden Flower* (1931), p. 35 and in Eva Wong's *Tales of the Dancing Dragon: Stories of the Tao* (2007), p. 75.

235 "Sea of *Qì*" (*qìhǎi* 氣海) refers to *Rèn* 6, located 1.5 cun below the umbilicus on the anterior midline. *Qìhǎi* ("Sea of Qì") is traditionally understood as a primary reservoir of original and acquired *qì*, central to vitality, constitutional strength, and the regulation of breathing, digestion, and reproductive function.

236The omentum is a major anatomical structure of the human abdomen and consists of two primary components: the greater omentum and the lesser omentum. Both are formed from visceral peritoneum, the thin serous membrane that lines the abdominal cavity and envelops the abdominal organs. The greater omentum is a large, apron-like fold that descends from the greater curvature of the Stomach, draping anteriorly over the small intestines. It then folds back on itself to attach to the transverse colon and the posterior abdominal wall. As a result of this folding pattern, the greater omentum is classically described as consisting of four layers of peritoneum formed by the doubled sheet that descends and then returns upward. The lesser omentum is thinner and more compact. It extends from the lesser curvature of the Stomach and the proximal duodenum to the Liver, anchoring these structures to the inferior surface of the diaphragm and posterior abdominal wall. Although smaller, it is continuous with the greater omentum as part of the overall peritoneal system. Within this region lies the epiploic (omental) foramen, an opening that permits the circulation of peritoneal fluid and communication between compartments of the peritoneal cavity.

From a *tàijí* and internal-cultivation perspective, it is often stated that abdominal breathing directed toward the *dāntián* 丹田 produces a gentle internal "massage" of the abdominal organs. This description reflects somatic and experiential observations used in cultivation traditions rather than an explicitly anatomical claim. A classical textual point of interest appears in the *Huángdì Nèijīng Sùwèn* 《黃帝內經素問》, Chapter 39, which discusses the "Sea of Qì" (*qìhǎi* 氣海) in relation to the *mó yuán* 膜原 ("membrane origin"). In his footnotes, Zhāng Zhìcōng 張志聰 (1619–1674) explains *mó yuán* as "the fatty membrane attached to the intestines and the Stomach." Classical sources further note that this tissue has a yellow coloration, consistent with adipose membranes.

Based on this description, some modern interpreters, including Professor Cheng, propose that *Mó Yuán* may correspond anatomically to the base of the omentum, and by extension may relate functionally to the *dāntián* as a visceral center. This identification, however, cannot be definitively confirmed and should be understood as an interpretive anatomical correlation, not an explicit statement made in the classical text itself.

237 In some Western medical texts, the omentum is referred to as the "policeman of the abdomen." It supports immunity through the production of milky spots, which are clusters of macrophages, and is known to isolate wounds and infections. The omentum helps limit the spread of intraperitoneal infections and can sometimes be observed encircling areas of trauma or infection. See Wang et al. (2020), *A Vibrant and Enigmatic Immunologic Organ Involved in Injury and Infection Resolution.*

---

[238] We can also recognize the "three *dāntián*" (*sān dāntián* 三丹田), which may be understood in relation to the three "ancestral" (*zōng* 宗) structures. The *zōng jīn* 宗筋 ("ancestral sinews") are located in the lower abdomen; the *zōng qì* 宗氣 ("ancestral *qì*") located in the chest; and the *zōng mài* 宗脈 ("*ancestral vessel*") associated with the region between the eyes. See Larre & Rochat de la Vallée (2003), *The Extraordinary Fu*, p. 57.

[239]"Greater Omentum" As a deliberate play on words, Professor Cheng records this term in his notes using a phonetic Chinese transliteration , writing it as *gé léi tè wūméntún* 葛雷特屋門屯. In this rendering, *gé léi tè* approximates the sound of "greater", while *wūméntún* approximates "omentum." The resulting characters, when translated literally in Chinese can be glossed as something like "special gray gate place," a meaning that is perhaps incidental rather than intended.

[240]"Lesser Omentum." In a similar phonetic and pedagogical manner, Professor Cheng renders this term in his notes as *lēi sài wūméntún* 勒賽屋門屯. In this construction, *lēi sài* approximates the sound of "lesser," while *wūméntún* again approximates "omentum." When translated literally, the characters 勒賽 may be glossed as *lēi* "to restrain, bind, or contain" and *sài* "to compete or contest." Taken together with *wūméntún* 屋門屯 ("house / gate / enclosure"), this yields an incidental literal sense along the lines of a "gated container."

[241] At the time of writing this book, this is how Western medicine largely viewed and understood these anatomical regions. However, subsequent contemporary Western medical studies now recognize the omentum as a dynamic immunologic organ, playing an active role in protecting the peritoneal cavity. In addition to its physical capacity to limit the spread of intraperitoneal infection, the omentum has been shown to orchestrate immune cell recruitment, particularly macrophages and mast cells, which participate in innate immune defense against internal infection. This expanded understanding aligns more closely with Professor Cheng's functional interpretation that emphasized responsiveness, containment, and internal regulation rather than passive anatomy alone. See Zareie, et al. (2006). *Novel Role for Mast Cells in Omental Tissue Remodeling and Cell Recruitment in Experimental Peritoneal Dialysis.*

242 Lesser Omentum as *Huángtíng* : the lesser omentum is a double layer of peritoneal tissue that extends from the Liver to the lesser curvature of the Stomach (hepatogastric ligament) and the first part of the duodenum (hepatoduodenal ligament). Above it attaches to the underside of the diaphragm. In Chinese history, The "Yellow Court" was considered the central meeting place in the Emperor's palace where his ministers gathered to discuss the regulation of the empire. The yellow color indicates Earth elemental phase (Spleen/Stomach) as the central organizing principle of the Five phase (*wǔxíng* 五行) arrangement with the four walls of the chamber representing the other four phases Wood (Liver), Fire (Heart), Metal (Lung), Water (Kidneys). Anatomically one might say that the lesser omentum – *Huángtíng* membranous space connects to the Stomach (Earth) in center of abdomen, to diaphragm with Lung (Metal) and Heart (Fire) above, to Liver (Wood) on the right, and Kidney (Water) below. It connects through the peritoneal lining of the Stomach with the greater omentum (*dāntián*) below.

243 The *Huáng Dì Nèijīng* 《黃帝內經》 medical texts date back to the Han Dynasty (206 BCE-220 CE) though many of the principles laid out in these texts have their origins during the 4th to 3rd centuries BCE when (as Paul Unschuld notes in the prologue to his translation) "*a new view on nature emerged in China. Comparable to the emergence of a science in the eastern Mediterranean only a few hundred years earlier, some Chinese philosophers began to perceive regularities in the daily workings of the universe that appeared to be governed by natural laws rather than numinous beings such as gods, ancestors, or ghosts.*" Unschuld & Tessenow (2011), p. 10.

244 Warring States period of China (475-221 BCE) was a period when Lǎozǐ 老子, Zhuāngzǐ 莊子 and Kǒngzǐ 孔子 (Confucius) lived.

Chapter 10: The Physiology of a Baby
嬰兒之生理[245]

In the *Huáng Dì Nèijīng* 《黃帝內經》 *(Yellow Emperor's Internal Medicine Classic) Qíbó* 岐伯[246] says: *"The sages arranged yin and yang [in such a way that their] sinews and vessels were in harmony, [their] bones and marrow were solid and firm, and [their] qi and blood both followed each other."*[247]

Lǎozǐ 老子 says in *Dàodé jīng* chapter 10:

專氣致柔能嬰兒乎

"In concentrating your qi and making it pliant, are you able to become (like) the newborn babe?"[248]

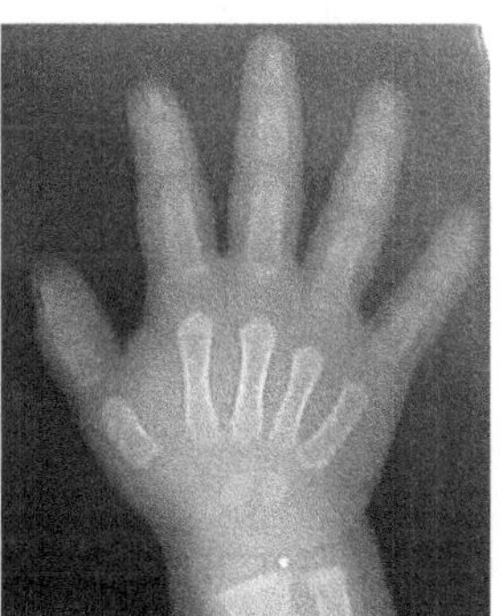

Figure 26: Normal X-Ray of a Young Child's Hand[249]

Source: Dr. Cowan's Patient Records

Now, with the help of this picture, I will explain the principles of the sages through physiological evidence. By examining the X-ray of the hand, one will notice the difference between the skeleton of a child and that of an adult.[250] The bones of a child appear to be separated far apart at every joint. What holds them together at these junctures is the network of ligaments, tendons and blood vessels, which act as flexible connections that facilitate movement.[251] Thus we can see that harmony of ligaments, tendons and blood vessels gives utmost benefit to movement. When qi and blood are full (and flowing), the entire body is like a rubber ball. A young child may fall to the ground, yet no harm is done to its body because the bones and marrow are firm and strong. This is what *Lǎozǐ* meant by "concentrate qi to attain pliancy."[252] It is hopeful that even the elderly, if they can learn how to circulate qi and blood, will regain this resilience and youthful rejuvenation.[253] It is indeed possible to master this exquisite principle without a doubt.

Ch. 10 Notes

---

245 *Shēnglǐ* 生理, ("Physiology"); "Life patterns": *Shēng* 生 – "life" or "birth," the same *shēng* as in the generating cycle of the Five Phases. *Lǐ* 理 – "principle, logic, internal pattern" is the same *lǐ* as in *zhélǐ* 哲理 ("sage principle," see Chapter 1) and *Lǐ, Qì, Xiàng* 理氣象 (see Chapter 3).

---

246 Qíbó 岐伯 is the legendary physician who advises the Yellow Emperor in the *Huáng Dì Nèijīng* 《黃帝內經》 (*Internal Medicine Classic* or the "Inner Classic").

247 *Huáng Dì Nèijīng Sùwèn* 《黃帝內經素問》, Chapter 3 "*Discourse on how Generative Qi communicates with Heaven*" (生氣通天論) the full quote is "*The sages arranged yin and yang [in such a way that their] sinews and vessels were in harmony, [their] bones and marrow were solid and firm, and [their] qi and blood both followed [their usual course]. In such a situation, inner and outer are balanced in harmony; an evil cannot cause harm; ears and eyes are clear; the qi set-up is as usual*" Unschuld & Tessenow (2011), p. 75.

248 Ames and Hall, (2003). *Dao De Jing: A Philosophical Translation* p. 90. An alternative translation by Red Pine simply reads "*Can you make your breath as soft as a baby's?*" Pine (1996) *Lao-tzu's Taoteching*, p. 20.

249 In the papers of Professor Cheng's medical discourses, we found a tiny X-ray of a child's hand that he apparently had been inspecting with his ever-present curiosity. Because of the poor quality of the original X-ray, we've replaced it with a clearer image to illustrate his point.

250 See the following Chapter 11: The Adult Skeleton.

251 The anatomic area of the wrist described by Professor Cheng here in the infant's X-ray is called the "growth plate" which is a highly active, vascularized region that has not yet calcified and therefore does not show up on X-ray (radiologic imaging does not pick up cartilage, ligaments, tendons and blood vessels). The wrist X-ray in children is commonly used to assess "bone age" by measuring the "space" between the bones as the wrist bones are not ossified at birth and maturation typically advances from the centers of ossification until puberty.

252 It is interesting to note that in East Asian medicine, *Yuán* 原 (source) translates as: "origin," "original," "beginning," "source," and refers to primordial qi as well as specific acupoints clustered around the wrist and ankles. These are the first acupoints mentioned in *Língshū* 《靈樞》 (*Spiritual* Pivot) Chapter 1, and are essential in promoting healthy growth and development throughout the body by accessing "primordial, original" *yuán* qi. Source points are commonly used in acupuncture for tonification, to improve blood circulation, warmth and vitality. Ed and I have discussed the *tàijí* practice of maintaining relaxed wrist and hands, the so called "beautiful lady's hand" in this context.

253 As stated earlier, according to the classics, qi is said to move the blood and blood carries the qi. They exist as an intimate *yīn-yáng* relationship.

Chapter 11: The Adult Skeleton
成人骨骼

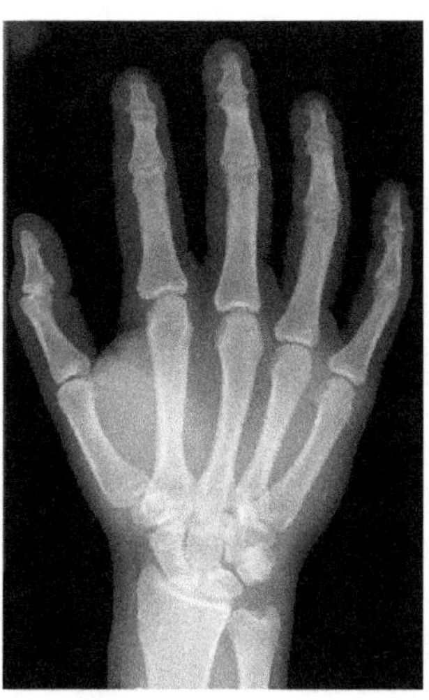

Figure 27: X-Ray of a Normal Adult Hand
Source: Dr. Cowan's Patient Records

In the X-ray of the adult skeleton one can see that the bones are tightly connected at every joint, exactly the opposite of a child.[254] This indicates that as one ages, the tendons become stiff due to poor circulation and loss of harmony between blood and qi .[255]

Furthermore, when the bones and marrow are subject to daily wear and tear, they lose their strength and firmness, falling into a state of deterioration. The bones become hard and brittle and cannot be compared with the child's softness and resiliency.

This is why *Lǎozǐ* says in Chapter 76:

堅強者死之徒 柔弱者生之徒
"The hard and rigid are companions of death.
The supple and soft are companions with life"[256]

Ch. 11 Notes

---

[254] See previous Chapter 10

[255] Improving loss of harmony between blood and qi with *Tàijí "Twenty-seven meta-analyses were synthesized in this scoping review with the aim of summarizing the current knowledge of the effectiveness of Tai Chi on health promotion of older adults. "High" and "moderate" quality evidence indicates that practicing Tai Chi can lead to significant improvements in balance, cardiorespiratory fitness (forced vital capacity and peak oxygen uptake), cognition (global cognition and executive function), mobility, proprioception, sleep and strength, as well as significant reductions in the incidence of falls and nonfatal stroke and reduction in stroke risk factors"* (Yang, et al. (2021), *Effectiveness of Tai Chi for Health Promotion of Older Adults: A Scoping Review of Meta-Analyses).*

Tàijí 太極 has specifically been shown to improve bone mineral density in middle aged and older adults, particularly in the lumbar spine. See Cui, Qian, & Liu (2025), *Effect of Tai Chi on Bone Mineral Density in Middle-Aged and Older Adults: A Meta-Analysis*.

[256] Ames & Hall (2003) *Dao De Jing: A Philosophical Translation*, p. 195.

Chapter 12: Explanation of the Sacrum 尾閭骨之解釋[257]

The sacrum and coccyx form the lowest part of the vertebral column. The sacrum consists of five fused vertebrae and is roughly wedge-shaped. It has eight openings assembled in two rows. The Chinese call it a *lǘ* 閭[258] or "lobby" in the sense that it serves as an entryway through a number of doors. The functions of these eight openings are most important and are considered strategic centers of physiological functioning, which should not be treated lightly. See Figure 28 below.

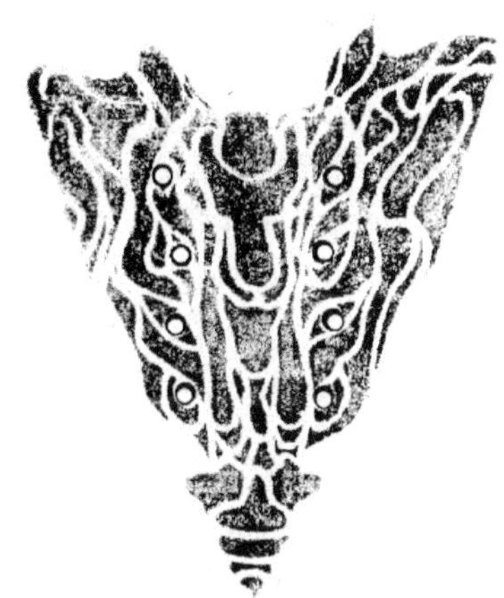

Figure 28: The Sacrum and Coccyx with the Eight Passageways
Illustration by Ed Young

These eight openings conduct essence-qi (*jīngqì* 精氣) from the *dāntián* 丹田 into the spinal column, called the "first pass,"[259] where it gradually condenses into marrow (*suǐ* 髓). From there, *jīngqì* passes up through the spine to the atlas vertebra ("Jade Pillow," *yù zhěn* 玉枕)[260] upon which the skull rests. This is "the second pass." It finally reaches the top of the brain (*níwán* 泥丸),[261] where the "soft spot" (posterior fontanelle) is located in infancy, this being the "third pass." The function of these three passes, and of the *jīngqì* and marrow has been described in Chapter 5 on *jīngqì* transformation, so I shall not repeat it here.

In my opinion, what is considered by Western medical science as important, such as blood circulation and internal secretions, is not nearly as important as the East Asian medical theory of transformation of *jīng* into *jīngqì*. According to *Cunningham's Textbook of Anatomy*, a standard medical text used in the West, the chapter on the sacrum begins with the sentence: *"The sacrum was at one time supposed to be the seed from which the body would be resurrected."*[262]

According to Webster's *Third New International Dictionary*, "resurrection" means *"the act or fact of rising again from a lower state of existence (as death, decay, disuse) to a superior state."*[263] Thus, the importance of the sacrum was once considered "sacred" by both Chinese and early Western medical sciences. It is a pity that the deeper meaning of the physiology of the sacrum seems to have been considered something mystical and therefore abandoned by Western medicine. It is a great loss to the study of human physiology and I hope that future generations of medical experts will give more serious attention to it.[264]

Ch. 12 Notes

---

257 *Wěi guān gǔ zhī jiěshì* 尾関骨之解釋: Literally, "Explanation of the Tail-bone Gate." The *weiguan gǔ* 尾関骨 is considered an important area in *tàijí* and *qìgōng* practice. See Appendix III: *Etymological Glossary of Sage Principle Terms*, for a more detailed analysis of these characters.

258 *Lǘ* 閭: A corridor, hallway, lobby, passageway, or rooms around the hall. This is the same character used in Chapter 6, where Professor Cheng plays on the English word "lumen." Example: *lǘ mén* 閭門, literally, a "lobby gate" or "hallway door."

259 "First Pass" (*yī kāi*一開) - In *tàijí* and *qìgōng* practice, there are considered three "passes" (*kāi*) along the spinal column that represent narrow gateways or passes that essence-qi (*jīngqì* 精氣) must move through in the process of transformation into *shén* 神 (spirit/consciousness).

260 "Jade Pillow" (*yù zhěn* 玉枕) is a Daoist term referring to the 2nd pass at the base of the skull. It is also the name for the related acupuncture point Bladder 9 on either side of the occipital protuberance of the skull.

261 *Níwán* 泥丸 literally "mudball" is an area at the top of the head known as the "third pass" that is thought to be related to acupuncture point Du 20 (*bǎi huì* 百會) "hundred meeting point."

262 While we could not find the quote in *Cunningham's Textbook on Anatomy* (1964) it is worth noting that the text is now in its 16th edition and has been extensively updated since the version cited by Professor Cheng, and the quote no longer appears in modern editions. However, there was a review article published in the Journal of the American Medical Association that states: *"The os sacrum (sacred bone) was so named by the Romans as a direct translation from the older Greek hieron osteon. Explanations of the attribute "sacred" or "holy" in the past have included misinterpretation of the Greek word hieron, use of the bone in sacrificial rites, the role of the bone in protecting the genitalia (themselves considered sacred), and the necessity for the intactness of this bone as a nidus for resurrection at the Day of Judgment. A more plausible explanation may be that the holiness of the sacral bone was an attribute borrowed from the ancient Egyptians, who considered this bone sacred to Osiris, the god of resurrection and of agriculture."* Kircher (1987). *How the sacrum got its name.*

263 Webster's *Third New International Dictionary*, published in September 1961. A newer edition of Webster's dictionary defines "resurrection" as "the revitalization or revival of something" which fits with Professor Cheng's deep interest in promoting qi transformation, quite literally "revitalization" in a person through *tàijí* medicine. It's also interesting to consider "resurrection" in the context of human evolution, as our capacity to stand up on two feet and see the horizon.

---

264 In this chapter we get another glimpse of Professor Cheng's earnest exploration of Western medical texts in an effort to connect East Asian medical principles with modern Western anatomic texts. The West currently tends to view the sacrum in strictly structural terms: The sacroiliac joint functions to absorb all the forces of the upper body before balancing and transferring the weight to the hips and legs. However, Professor Cheng asks us to consider the deeper, as yet, unrecognized physiological functions of this structure beyond the bone. One wonders what Professor Cheng would have thought of the work in *Craniosacral Osteopathy,* by Dr. William Sutherland (1873-1954), who recognized the hidden functions of the sacrum in promoting health by way of the refined rhythms of circulation of cerebral spinal fluid. Sutherland said "one must visualize the movement of the sacrum and the ilia as having two distinct features: the postural movement of the greater part of the sacroiliac joint on the auricular surfaces and the involuntary *respiratory* movement of the sacrum between the ilia allowed by the change in the divergence of the articular faces." It was this so-called "respiratory movement" that Sutherland said lies *"within the cerebrospinal fluid [where] there is an invisible element that I refer to as the 'Breath of Life.'"* Magoun (1976). *Osteopathy in the Cranial Field,* p. 34. This description of the "breath of life" through the membranes comes remarkably close to the East Asian concept of *qì* 氣 (breath).

Chapter 13: The Mystery of Hormones 荷爾蒙之究竟[265]

The mystery and wonder of hormones have been repeatedly cited in Western medical journals. A hormone has been described as a chemical manufactured by the cells of endocrine glands and tissues affecting organ function. These chemical messengers are also said to occur from the endings of nerve cells and transmitted to other nerve cells.[266] No one has as yet offered a complete explanation of the causes of hormonal action, only explaining the extraordinary effects. Although I dare not claim complete understanding of Western medical endocrinology, I shall try to compare what classical Chinese medicine describes with what is already available in the West in order to perhaps throw some light upon the matter.

Production of hormones by approximately "fifteen glands" in the human body corresponds to the two circulatory systems, which East Asian medicine calls the *Rèn* vessel *(Rènmài* 任脈) and *Dū vessel* (*Dū mài* 督脈)[267] and what Daoist practitioners call the "Water Wheel Cycle,"[268] also known as the microcosmic orbit (see Figure 30).

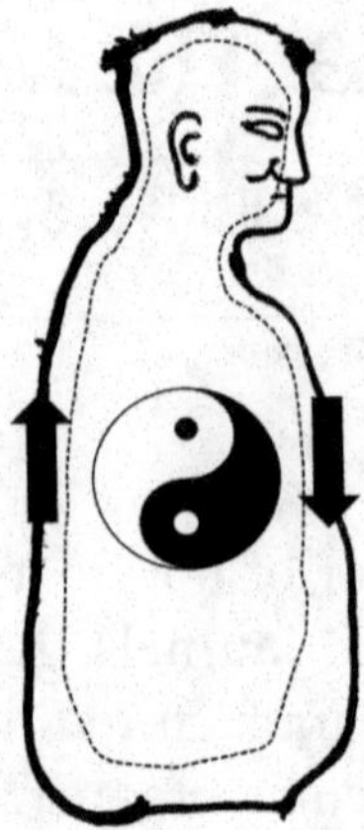

Figure 29: The Microcosmic Circulation
Illustration by Ed Young

Its function will be explained according to East Asian medical principles for study by the Western medical field. The *Rènmài* and *Dūmài* and the "water wheel cycle" were previously described in Chapter 6 "*Jīngqì* 精氣," Chapter 8 "Heart and Spine" and Chapter 11 "the Sacrum" and won't be repeated here.

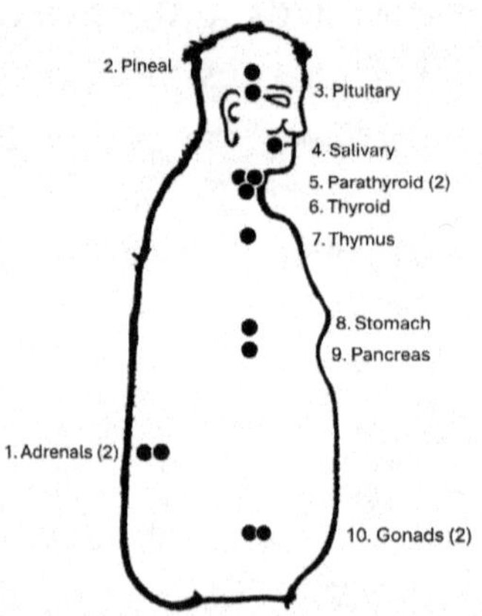

Figure 30: The Circulation of the Unified Hormonal System[269]
Illustration by Ed Young

For the sequence of the hormonal glands, primary importance should be given to the adrenal glands (see Figure 31):[270]

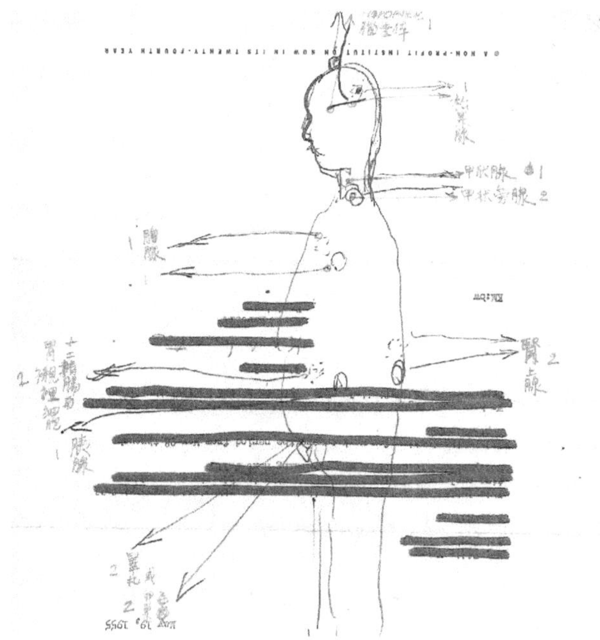

Figure 31: Professor Cheng's Rough Sketch of the 15 Glands[271]

1. The two adrenal glands are what the ancient *Book of Luo* refers to as "Heaven gives birth to Water."[272] In terms of the five phases (*wǔxíng* 五行), the Kidney-urogenital-adrenal system corresponds to the Water phase. *Jīngqì* 精氣 (urogenital essence-qi) is drawn up the spine (*Dū* vessel) through the first pass, the sacrum (see Chapter 12). As it ascends, it passes through the adrenal glands.
2. At the Atlas vertebra called "Jade Pillow" (*yùzhěn* 玉枕)[273] the pineal gland commands the second pass.[274]
3. The Pituitary gland[275] is near the third pass, called "the mud pellet" (*ní wán* 泥丸).[276]

4. When the *jīngqì* has crossed the third pass of the water wheel cycle, it combines with the saliva.[277]
5. The *jīngqì* then passes downward by way of the two salivary tracts that lie beneath the tongue and thus reaches the thyroid and parathyroid glands in the neck.
6. The *jīngqì* then passes from *Dū* to *Rèn* Vessel through the thymus gland called "the twelve story tower."[278]
7. It then passes through the pancreas and Stomach belonging to the Spleen network.[279]
8. From here the *jīngqì* passes down through the testes (male) and the ovaries (female) that represent the end of the *Rèn* vessel thus completing the fifteen glandular points.[280]

The sequence of circulation follows this order without deviating in the slightest way. Its passage from beginning to end is simply the source of the main course of internal secretions. The only differences between the Chinese and Western medicine are in perspectives and the terminology used.[281]

The Jīnyè 津液 Saliva as a Hormonal Secretion[282]

The bodily secretions differ in nature from one organ to another. The *jīng* 精 (essences) within each organ possess two qualities (*yīn-yáng* 陰陽).

One particular example is saliva which contains *yīn-yáng* aspects. *Jīn* has more *yáng* qualities and is produced by qi/breath whereas *yè* is more *yīn* and is produced by blood (*xuè* 血). On closer examination (of their *yīn-yáng* nature), each aspect of these secretions reveals its own unique sources, functions, order, beginning and ending. The knowledge of its functions gives it its name. *Jīn* 津 secretions are thin and travel along the windpipe (trachea), passing through the Lungs (as respiratory secretions) into the membranes and connective tissues (and into the blood). *Yè* 液 secretions are thicker and travel through the esophagus, entering the Stomach and then on to the five major *zàng* 臟 organ networks.[283] The two-character term *Jīnyè* is used for saliva to show that it has *yīn-yáng* qualities.

It is said that some hormones are excreted directly into the blood stream, while others take an indirect route into the blood and there are still other hormones that do not enter the blood stream at all but function locally. This differentiation is due to the relative *yīn-yáng* qualities in different hormones. Blood is considered *yīn* while qi is considered *yáng* in nature. Qi is carried by the blood along its route: thus a hormone can enter the blood stream directly or indirectly depending on its *yīn-yáng* affinities.[284] Furthermore, hormones that do not enter the blood directly have different transforming functions.[285]

The so-called "Golden Elixir" *jīnjīn yùyè*[286] in Daoist internal cultivation and East Asian medicine is considered one aspect of the major life force in the human body whose functions are comparable to transformative activities of other hormones. This is why I have brought up these two points (circulation of the hormones and importance of saliva) to explain the motive force of qi, the order of its passage, and the mutual relationships of hormones in their function. Since I find no inconsistencies between Western and East Asian medicine here, I have no doubt that we are considering the same subject from different points of view.[287]

The Use of Animal Hormones in Medicine

Hormones extracted from animals and plants are now being analyzed and used to supplement hormone deficiencies in humans. This method has arisen from advances in modern

Western science. While hormones from foreign sources may benefit human health, they may also violate natural physiological principles and can result in injury. We must study this subject exhaustively and responsibly.

Here are several points worth considering:

The human body is created by way of its own powers of production and regeneration.[288] If a deficiency is discovered, isn't it more logical to attempt to recover this innate regenerative power before considering the use of hormones from other species? Only when the body can no longer generate its own regenerative power, then introduction of a substitute as a supplement should be considered. If this possibility of regeneration is ignored, however, I would consider the rush to use hormone replacement from sources outside the human body an irresponsible healing practice.[289]

If a hormone is depleted in the human body, we will observe a person's qi (life-giving force) becoming visibly weakened. This symptom should be treated before it becomes life-threatening. However, if foreign hormones are introduced too quickly to replace the deficiency, it can lead to serious illness or even death. Why? Because the life-giving qi from one species is not the same as another. A depleted hormone cannot be replaced sufficiently this way because the different nature and proportions of *yīn-yáng* functions between species do not match up. This overly simplistic practice alone is inadequate treatment. The reason is that human hormones exist as part of a whole system and supplementing one hormone (by injection etc.) from an external (non-human) source can produce an excess that will create an imbalance (*yīn-yáng*) within the whole system of hormones in the body, thus suppressing other aspects of the hormonal system.[290] Disease can be caused by excess as much as by deficiency. If treating the deficiency is not done properly, the natural secretion of the fifteen (endocrine/exocrine) glands will be imbalanced causing the circulating hormones to lose their systematic function.[291] When, for example, a man is given a woman's hormone, his nature changes; he will develop breasts and male sex organs will shrink. When a woman is given male hormones, her nature changes as seen in the shrinking of her breasts and the growing of beard and whiskers. This is evidence of the relationship and proportion of *yīn-yáng* present in hormones. It also adds evidence to the importance of considering hormone balances as an integral part of "The Golden Elixir cultivation." The distribution of the Golden Elixir is as follows: the *jīn (*which is *yáng* in nature*)* reaches the six *fŭ* bowels (which are *yáng* in nature) and the *yè* (*yīn* in nature) enters the five *zàng* organs (which are *yīn* in nature.)[292] Together the *Jīnyè* secretions function to breakdown food essence (*jīng*), thus increasing the vitality essence-qi (*jīngqì*) in the bowels and organs, which is analogous to the stimulating effects of other hormones, thus making saliva (and other digestive secretions) an important part of the whole system of the fifteen hormonal glands. When the *jīng*-essences extracted from food and liquids of the bowels and organs are full, they overflow and are stored in the Kidneys (urogenital adrenal system). This then becomes the raw material that makes the Golden Elixir (*jīndān* 金丹) in men and women. Is this not the mystery and wonder of the whole system of hormones indeed marvelous?[293]

In truth, there is no other life-giving force in the human body that has such profound functions as hormones. East Asian medicine is based in the Sage principles. Neither exists without the other. All Chinese Sage principles are based on the principles of Nature (*yīn-yáng*), and the fundamental principles of Nature are indeed mysterious and complex, therefore difficult to describe. According to what has been stated in *The*

Science of Life,[294] the science of endocrinology and the study of hormones is still in its infancy. This important research is of much value and cannot help but evoke deep admiration.

Ch. 13 Notes

---

265 *Hé ĕr méng zhī jiū jìng* 荷爾蒙之究竟: Literally getting to the bottom of hormones. Hormone (*hè'ĕrméng* 荷爾蒙) is a borrowed transliterated word from English.

266 Professor Cheng's holistic understanding of hormonal secretion and neurotransmitters presents the nervous, endocrine, and exocrine systems as components of a single, integrated regulatory network. This unified perspective, once considered unconventional, is increasingly reflected in contemporary Western medicine. As stated in Malcolm J. Low in *Williams Textbook of Endocrinology* (2016): "*The field of neuroendocrinology has expanded from its original focus on the control of pituitary hormone secretion by the hypothalamus to encompass multiple reciprocal interactions between the central nervous system (CNS) and endocrine systems in the control of homeostasis and physiologic responses to environmental stimuli* " pp. 109-175. This evolution in neuroendocrinology underscores the growing recognition of the dynamic and reciprocal relationships among these systems.

267 *Rèn and Dū* have already been discussed in previous chapters. See Appendix III: *Etymological Glossary of Sage Principle Terms*, for a more detailed analysis of *mài* 脈.

268 "Water Wheel Cycle" *héchē dǎoyùn* 河車倒運 literally: "Water wheel reverse cycle."

Daniel Schrier, editor: The "waterwheel" (*héchē* 河車) appears in the *Nèijīng Tú* 《內經圖》 (*Map of the Inner Landscape*), illustrating the microcosmic orbit, also known as the lesser celestial circuit (*xiǎo zhōu tiān* 小周天). This diagram maps the circulation of celestial energy within the body. The microcosmic orbit is a foundational practice of "inner alchemy" (*nèidān* 內丹) involving the refinement and circulation of vital essence. Energy ascends along the Governing Vessel (*dū mài*) and descends along the Conception Vessel (*rèn mài*), forming a continuous loop. Through this circulation, the body becomes an integrated whole, a "ring" (*huán* 環). This dynamic movement supports the awakening of the subtle body and, when combined with sustained cultivation of stillness, it facilitates the profound integration and internal transformation of body, mind, and spirit.

269 Illustration by Ed Young based on a quick sketch Professor Cheng made for this book.

270 Adrenal gland (*shèn shàng* 腎上) literally: "above the Kidney" is analogous to the English "Ad-Renal." Anatomically, the adrenal glands sit on top of the Kidneys and are considered in the *Nèijīng* medical classics to be within the realm of the urogenital or Kidney organ network associated with the Water phase. This area along the back also relates to the so called "gate of life" (*mìng mén* 命門 associated with acupuncture point Du 4 that is located at the level of the second lumbar vertebra right between the two Kidneys).

271 This quick sketch of the 15 glands was found in Professor's papers. He apparently created it to explain the principle of the 15 glands to Ed Young and Tam Gibbs back when he was writing the Sage Principles.

272 "Heaven first gives birth to Water" (*tiān yīshēng shuǐ* 天一生水). See Chapter 3 on the sequence of generation of the eight trigrams.

---

273 "The three gates or passes" (*guān* 關) described in the previous chapter. In Daoist cultivation practice this refers to the three places along the spine that represent difficult areas for primordial *jīngqì* to pass through. The "Jade Pillow" (*yùzhěn* 玉枕) is located at the posterior base of the occipital skull and is the name given to the bilateral acupuncture points Bladder 9 located in this area.

Daniel Schrier, editor: The *Nèijīng Tú* 《內經圖》 (*Map of the Inner Landscape*), an alchemical map of the body, depicts the "Three Passes" or "energetic gates" (*sān guān* 三關). These are critical spiritual and energetic gateways located along the spinal column, forming a pathway that connects the lower abdomen to the cranial region. Each pass represents a stage in the practitioner's meditative ascent toward internal alchemical transformation. This pathway mirrors the flow of qi in meditation practices, particularly the "Lesser Celestial Circuit" (*xiǎo zhōu tiān* 小周天), in which energy circulates through the Governing Vessel (*dū mài* 督脈) and the Conception Vessel (*rèn mài* 任脈). The "Upper Pass" or "Jade Pillow" (*yùzhěn* 玉枕), is positioned at the base of the skull and symbolizes spiritual ascent and enlightenment. This pass corresponds with the acupuncture point *nǎohù* 腦戶 (Brain's Door; Du 17).

274 The pineal gland is anatomically located in the midline of the brain behind the third ventricle at the top of the brainstem. It has a curious structure partially resembling a "third eye" and plays a central role in regulating circadian rhythms through its production of melatonin. In the Chinese medicine classics, the sage is said to stay aligned with the circadian cycles of Nature (the macrocosm of day/night) in order for one's metabolic microcosm to be healthy. This is exemplified by the ancient Chinese phrase *tiān rén hé yī* 天人合一 which means "the heavens (Nature) and human are one." The first chapter of the *Huáng Dì Nèijīng* 黃帝內經 (Yellow Emperor Internal Medicine Classic) states the importance of living aligned with the cycles of Nature: "*The sages lived in harmony with heaven and earth and followed the patterns of the eight winds*" (Unschuld and Tessenow (2011), p. 43). It's also worth noting that there are a number of acupuncture pointes clustered around the back of the skull called are "wind" points that protect against invasion of cold wind, which is why Professor Cheng always advised to protect one's neck from cold drafts.

275 The pituitary gland is the pea-sized gland located centrally at the base of the brain. It produces a number of hormones critical to the regulation of body functions.

---

276 *Níwán gōng* 泥丸宮 (mud ball palace) is an alternative name given to acupoint Du 20 located at the top of the head (Ellis & Wiseman (1989), *Grasping the Wind: An Exploration into the Meaning of Chinese Acupuncture Point Names* p. 343).

Daniel Schrier, editor: In Daoist alchemical practice, the *Níwán gōng* (泥丸宮), or "Palace of Nirvana," resides in the upper elixir field (*dāntián* 丹田). It usually refers to the center of the head or the crown point and appears in Daoist internal cultivation diagrams such as the *Nèijīng Tú* 《內經圖》 (*Map of the Inner Landscape*) and the *Xiūzhēn Tú* 《修真圖》 (*Map for Cultivation of Reality*). The head is considered the heavenly part of the body and the celestial origin of the individual. It contains layers of celestial realms as well as the processes required to transcend physical existence. The forehead and nose areas in these diagrams are labeled with the names of deities, celestial locations, and internal energetic sites, including the Muddy Pellet (*níwán* 泥丸) and the Celestial Eye (*tiān mù* 天目) located between the eyes. The Muddy Pellet (*níwán* 泥丸) is associated with the physical root of the pineal gland and is described as having nine cavities, corresponding to the Nine Heavenly Palaces (*jiǔxiāo* 九霄). These symbolize progressive stages on the path toward spiritual immortality through the alignment and refinement of one's *yuánshén* 元神 (Original Spirit).

277 Saliva: *jīnjīn yùyè* 金津玉液 "golden nectar" literally: gold spring jade fluid: In contrast to Western endocrinology, Professor Cheng includes the salivary glands as a key component of the unified hormonal circulatory system rather than merely an unrelated part of the digestive secretion. (See below for more on saliva as a hormone.)

278 Thymus (*xiongxian* 胸腺): literal "chest gland" According to modern East Asian medical terminology, this corresponds to the thymus. The "twelve-story tower" *shí èr chóng lóu*十二重楼 refers the segmented, ringed structure of the trachea. It evokes the image of a tower or pagoda with twelve stacked sections, symbolized as a channel, both for receiving air/breath/qi and activating the *Jīngqì* 精氣 (now present in the saliva) and transfer of the "Golden Nectar"(*jīnjīn)* into the *Rèn* vessel (called "the Conception Vessels." The thymus gland is responsible for producing and maturing T-cell lymphocytes, critical for long-term memory in the immune system, which help fight infections. In children, the thymus gland is quite large and can fill half the chest, a reflection of the intensely active immune-learning process a child must go through in adapting to the world. At its base, the thymus is anatomically related to the Heart and Lungs and at its apex with the mouth and tongue.

279 The glands of the Stomach form a sophisticated network divided into three parts, each producing different hormones important for digestion, which Professor Cheng includes as part of the unified hormonal system rather than being relegated to the digestive system alone. The pancreas is a complex structure of both endocrine and digestive (exocrine) hormones that corresponds to one aspect of the Spleen network (*pí* 脾) corresponding to the Earth phase in East Asian medicine.

280 According to Professor Cheng's sketch of the unified hormonal system, there are 15 active glands: 2 adrenal, 1 pituitary, 1 pineal, 1 thyroid, 2 parathyroid, 1 thymus, 1 Stomach, 1 pancreas, 2 salivary and 2 testes/2 ovaries.

281 Here Professor presents his holistic view of the endocrine/exocrine system as linked in one communicating (water-wheel) cycle whereas Western medicine organizes the endocrine organs into separate parts.

282 *Jīnyè* 津液 is a Chinese medical term for digestive secretions or body fluids in general. Professor here includes the circulation of the *Jīnyè*, demonstrating in their *yīn-yáng* functions in the body which reflect the sage principles found in the Unschuld (2016) *Huang Di Nei Jing Ling Shu: The ancient classic on needle therapy*. Chapter 36, p. 385.

283 The *yè* 液 are specifically mentioned in the title of *Língshū* 《靈樞》 Chapter 28: as having "*the special conduction and transmission of the yè liquids to the top of the body at the level of the eyes. The eyes are presented as the place where a lot of the vital circulation accumulates and because all this network of animation comes together in this place, the yè , the concentrated, dense, bodily liquid, goes up to that area and the brain*" Larre & Rochat de la Vallée (2003), *The Extraordinary Fu*, p. 48.

284 A fundamental principle of *Yìjīng* 《易經》 based East Asian medicine is that *yīn* has an affinity for *yáng* and *yáng* has an affinity for *yīn*. Neither can exist purely on its own.

285 "Hormones that do not enter the blood…" Professor Cheng seems to be making an important distinction between the Endocrine and Exocrine glands. Exocrine glands secrete their substances locally through ducts onto cell surfaces. Examples are tears, sweat, saliva, breast milk, and digestive secretions. On the other hand, endocrine glands secrete their substances directly into the bloodstream. This is why they are called "ductless glands." Neurotransmitters and neurohormones secreted by the neuroendocrine cells of the hypothalamus are transported directly along nerves to the cells of the anterior pituitary and may be considered to indirectly enter the bloodstream.

286 "Golden Elixir" (*jīnjīnyùyè* 金津玉液) is a term used in Daoist cultivation practices (literally: "golden liquid and jade fluid.") In East Asian medicine, *jīnjīnyùyè* happens to be the name of an extra acupuncture point located underneath the tongue on the salivary glands on either side of the frenulum of the tongue that excretes saliva. During the Tang dynasty (618-907 CE), the great physician Sūn Sīmiǎo 孫思邈 (581-682 CE) indicated bleeding of these points for sudden swelling of the tongue, which obstructs breathing.

287 "Different points of view" meaning that when saliva is considered as part of the hormonal system we get a glimpse of a holistic system of *yīn-yáng* representing the mutual relationship of blood and qi in the body.

288 "Regenerative power" literally: "the power to transform life: (*huà shēng zhī lì* 化生之力) Though Professor Cheng may not have known this at the time, this "regenerative power" may perhaps be analogous to the current research into the activity of pluripotent stem cells currently being investigated as potential sources of regenerating organs.

289 Professor Cheng is cautioning against the rush to use hormone replacement derived from other animals before considering internal cultivation practices. At the time of the writing of this book, hormone replacement was being used with increasing frequency in Western medicine, e.g. insulin and thyroid hormone derived from pig etc. Currently synthetic hormones are being used in Western medicine quite frequently. One wonders what Professor Cheng would have thought about a hormone created in a lab.

290 Professor Cheng's understanding of the endocrine/exocrine secretions as a whole system is remarkable. It is now well understood in Western medicine that the addition of excessive external hormones can interfere with natural feedback loops of hormone production. For instance, the overuse of adrenal corticosteroids can result in adrenal insufficiency and risk of acute death. This illustrates a fundamental *yīn-yáng* principle of things pushed past their prime revert to their opposite

291 Professor Cheng is making an important point here that changing one hormone level can affect the balance and relationships of the endocrine/exocrine system when understood as a unified whole. This is rarely appreciated in western endocrinology.

292 In East Asian medicine, the six viscera/bowels (*fǔ* 腑) include the "hollow" organs, Stomach, small intestine, large intestine, bladder, gall bladder and are considered *yáng* in nature relative to the five solid organs (*zàng* 臟), Spleen, Heart, Lung, Kidney, Liver that are considered more *yīn*.

293 Professor Cheng is pointing out the primary role of saliva in the processes now understood to be the unified neuro-gastro-endocrine system. As noted in Cryan et al. (2018), *The Neuroendocrinology of the Microbiota–gut–brain Axis: A Behavioural Perspective* pp. 80-101.

---

[294] *The Science of Life,* is a three-volume work by H. G. Wells, Julian Huxley, and G. P. Wells, and was first published in 1929–30 by The Waverley Publishing Company and later revised as a single-volume edition in 1939 by Garden City Publishing Company. Intended as a comprehensive and accessible account of contemporary biological knowledge, it has been described as *"the first modern textbook of biology,"* Smith (1986). *H. G. Wells: Desperately mortal*, p. 263.

The Science of Life appears to have made a significant impression on Professor Cheng, particularly in affirming his ideas about East Asian medicine. Notably, it introduced the term "New Ecology" (p. 961), anticipating developments in ecological thought such as Arthur Tansley's 1935 formulation of the ecosystem concept. Later philosophical discussions of this ecological perspective appear in works such as Warwick Fox's article *Deep Ecology: A New Philosophy of Our Time?* (1984) and J. Baird Callicott's *Intrinsic Value, Quantum Theory, and Environmental Ethics* (1985), which explore the convergence and complementary features of what came to be called the "New Physics" and the "New Ecology."

It is this ecological vision, grounded in the interrelatedness of life which resonates with Professor Cheng's assertion that *"All Chinese Sage Principles are rooted in the principles of nature."*

End Note

In this book I have simply used the words of the Chinese sages from thousands of years ago to compare and contrast with what is currently known in Western medicine. It is my hope that medical experts in the West may find these Sage principles of some use in advancing their research and practice so that such profound wisdom will not be lost to the ages. May communication between Eastern and Western medicine bring people good health around the world.

Cheng, Man-ching
New York, 1972

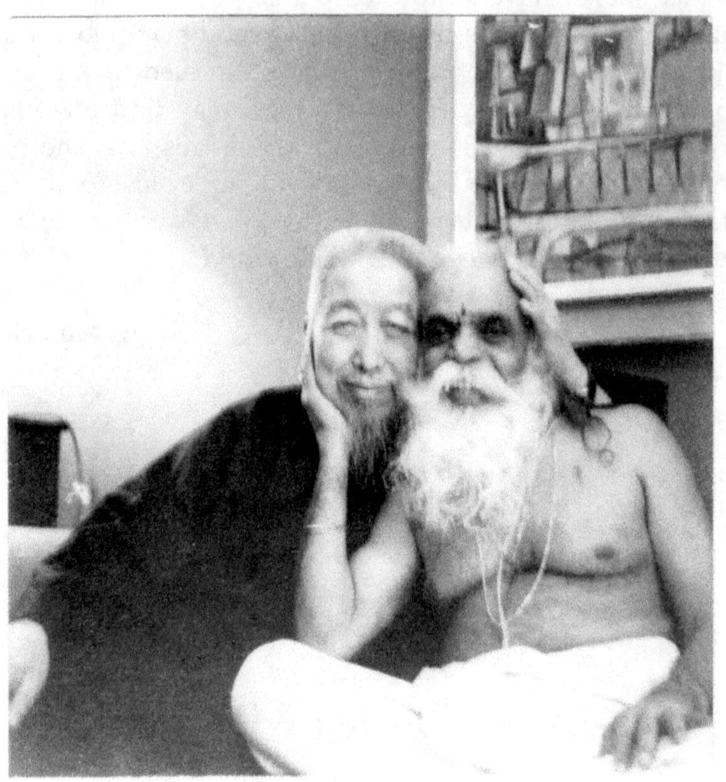

Professor Cheng with Swami Bua[295]

[295] Unknown date and photographer

Appendix I: Parting Words of Professor Cheng from January 1974, Six Chinese Characters of Health 大欲 飲食 起處[296]

Six Chinese Characters of Health
dà yù yǐn shí qǐ chǔ 大欲飲食起處

This is a very lucky day today. To have Swami Bua come and talk with us this way is a very rare occasion.[297] I understand a few points of what Swami was talking about, and they have much in common with the Chinese conception of health. For example, when people are young and healthy, they can see well in the dark and yet in old age, night vision is poor. This simply means that your light is no longer strong enough.

In terms of physical movement, "external" types of exercise do not use very much qi. They depend on the forceful movement the muscles themselves and not the movement of qi. For instance, in meditation, you have the movement of internal energy (qi) and yet the body itself does not move very much. There are two sides to movement, *yīn-yáng*, which are like two sides of a coin, front and back. In actual fact, both sides are very important. In certain regards, exercise is looked upon in the same way the world over.

What I want to speak about here today to my fellow students is the Chinese concept of health. Human health can in no case be separated from the physiology of the body. If one were to speak of health as if it were separate from physiology, it would be merely a matter of fighting. Now, China has many types of exercises too, the martial arts, so to speak. But what I want to discuss today, what is most important, is the unifying theme of health and physiology. In this regard I bring up six

Chinese characters that relate to the primary goals of good health:

- Great Desire (sexual relations) (*dà yù* 大欲)
- Drinking and Eating (*yǐn shí* 飲食)
- Getting up in the morning and settling down at night (*qǐ chǔ* 起處)

Now the first four characters Great Desire (*dà yù* 大欲) and Drinking and Eating (*yǐn shí* 飲食) over the past million years have obviously been very important for our health and survival. Now add two more characters: *qǐ chǔ* 起處; the first, *qǐ*, means getting up early and going out and doing activities and the second, *chǔ* means coming back home after doing our work, settling down and getting a good night of sleep.

yǐn shí 飲食 (eating and drinking)

Why do we not just say "eating?" Why is there one word for drinking and another for eating? The difference between these two characters is very important. Chinese medical theory is based on *yīn-yáng* dynamics and here in *tàijí* practice we speak about these two off-setting each other as complementary principles. An example is the sun. Now if you consider the plants and animals in Nature, if there were to be unending sunshine, plants and animals would burn up. And if there were no sun, only moon, all life would freeze. So this is an example of how *yīn-yáng* must mutually nurture life.[298] This is why we say in *tàijí* 太極, that *yīn* must never leave *yáng* and *yáng* must never leave the *yīn*. They co-respond, complementing each other, like front and back, top and bottom.

So now when we look at these characters for eating and drinking, if it was only one without the other, it would not support health. During the Zhou dynasty,[299] these two characters were used to imply good health: eating means taking in substantial food to nourish the *yáng* side of our physiology and drinking (tea, water, soup, wine) nourishes the *yīn* side. In the same way, sleeping at night nourishes the *yīn* side while rising up and being active during the day nourished the *yáng* side of our life. Not sleeping at night is like the plants burning when there's too much sun. From a (*yīn-yáng*) physiological perspective, lack of sleep dries us up. That is why we must always have a proper balance of both complements, *yīn-yáng*. In the same manner, in our diet, proper hydration is just as important as food for good health. For example, if someone has an illness, no matter how severe it may be, there is always a way to treat it. Now we all possess an important oral secretion, saliva (*jīn yè*),[300] but if that becomes deficient in someone who is seriously ill, no matter how much medicine they receive, they will not recover. From an East Asian medicinal perspective, when someone is ill, the most essential thing to do is to nourish the *yīn* with fluids. This is why, in the Chinese character pair for diet, drinking (*yǐn* 飲) comes first.[301]

Besides food and drink, I would like to speak about movement as it pertains to our health. Rest and activity, like drinking and eating make a complementary *yīn-yáng* pair. For example, if we are always active, moving around, never still, we deplete our qi, the *yáng* side of our physiology, and this will eventually hurt the *yīn*.[302] If we are a little more restful, take it easy and don't overdo the active life, then gradually the vitality of *yīn* will return. Once you understand how these two complementary aspects of our physiology function together, you will have something that can be put into practical use immediately to support your health.

For example, here we are, talking a lot. If you are ever in a situation like this, remember from time to time to take a breath of air (*qì* 氣) all the way down to your abdomen. This will regulate your system so that you won't deplete your qì and dry yourself out. No matter where you are or what time it may be, if you feel yourself becoming too tired or too overworked, that same method of "swallowing a mouthful of air (*qì*)"[303] can restore your physical and mental vitality. When talking for a long time, if your mouth feels dry just let your tongue touch the top of your palate and move it around a little bit and it will produce saliva to moisten your mouth (*yīn* supporting *yáng*). Swallow this saliva down to your *dantian*.[304] This is the same as drinking a cup of soup or having a drink of water to revitalize the *yīn* part of your physiology. It is a very simple yet practical way for you to put into practice some of the lessons in nourishing the *yīn* side of your metabolism to support your *yáng*.

I am not going to go into a more expanded discussion of these four characters, I am simply presenting this as a preliminary step in supporting your health. If I were to go into more depth, I think it would be too much for the translators to convey at this time. So again, I repeat, if you feel your mouth becoming dry, recognize that this is an excess of yang at the expense of yin and try swallowing a little bit of saliva and you will find that it immediately helps you feel more comfortable by reinforcing the *yīn* side of your health.

This question of food and drink is a vast and profound topic that cannot be finished in a short talk. An old friend of mine, Mr. Tu (Tu Hsin Wu),[305] I hear is still alive. He is still healthy at 160 years old! He would often scold people at the drop of a hat, no matter what their position or status, about their eating habits. He would ask, "Do you understand what food is all about?" In point of fact, most of us do not truly appreciate what eating is. We simply put food in our mouth, it tastes good, we chew it and swallow it, and that's it. But the real question about eating is much more profound, so I am using this opportunity to speak with my fellow students about eating and drinking as a simple method to support your health.

There is another old friend of mine, Wellington Xu, who is 92 years old and still healthy. He's like a monkey! We sit and talk together and he's always moving – sliding up and down in his chair and wiggling around. He never sits still! You would never be able to guess that he's 92 years old: his health is better than mine! It is truly something remarkable. I asked him what his method for staying healthy was, and this is what he told me. He said, "Eating and drinking is 50% of health. Once I take food in my mouth, I chew it many times, that's where I have control over it, because once I swallow it, I have no real control of how it will be metabolized. As long as I have it between my teeth, I am in charge of my digestion. You would do well to study this."

Now I have my own phrase to add to this. While there is only so much we can do to support our digestion, I feel certain my elder brother will feel that what I've said here is correct. "Eat Less!" Absolutely avoid overeating. This is the first thing to remember. The thing you enjoy the most, gradually cut down on it. Be especially certain that when you do see something that you really love and you know it is very rich, take it easy, take it slow, eat just a little bit. This is very, very, important! I cannot tell you how much I stress this. In reference to rich food, which is very heavy, this kind of food is the worst possible thing for your Stomach to process. Because it's so rich and heavy, you must eat only a small amount and really chew it well.

Second, there are three meals in a day: morning, noon, night. If it is not time to eat, avoid snacks. Eating between meals doesn't allow the Stomach time to rest properly.

Now here is something that you Americans will find very strange, indeed: chewing gum. Gum has many things in it that put out the (Stomach) fire. It has mint in it that is very cooling. This will reduce the Stomach's capacity to digest properly. Americans like to chew gum especially when they're dating; when boys and girls get close together they chew gum to keep their breath fresh and sweet. But when you suppress Stomach fire, that's the cause of bad breath to begin with! Here is an example of the universal *tàijí* principle: if you try to suppress something, it will eventually come back stronger. So actually, suppressing Stomach fire by chewing gum all day (or taking antacids) reduces it to a kind of smoldering embers that will actually build up its power and come back with a vengeance.[306] I am bringing this up as an important subject because those of you who often chew gum are hurting your Stomach metabolism by never letting it rest. In East Asian medicine we say that prenatal qi (*yuánqì* 元氣) depends on the Kidney network, but once we are born it is the Stomach (and Spleen) that we depend on to nourish our life. Whether we live to 100 or not, we are always going to depend on our Stomach, so we should put our strongest attention on how we treat it.

To go a little deeper, I would like to talk about the five phases (*wǔxíng* 五行) and five organ networks (*wǔzàng* 五臟). In terms of digestion, the Spleen and Stomach are a pair that work together like *yīn-yáng* respectively. The Spleen sits beside the Stomach and causes it to move and digest.[307] In East Asian medicine, we use a word to describe the nature of the Spleen and that is *xìn* 信 meaning 'trust' or 'sincerity.'[308] When you eat something, you fill the Stomach up and it sits there. The Spleen sits behind the Stomach and "kicks" it into action.[309] This is the sincerity and reliability of the Spleen to move things along in the digestive system. Therefore, it is so important to have set times to eat and to avoid eating too much in order to support the Spleen's function without overwhelming it. For example, if you are accustomed to eating two bowls of rice a day, then try to maintain this consistency rather than eating three bowls one day and one bowl the next. So, to repeat, eat less, reduce what you love the most, and eat at set times. This is how one supports the yin side (Spleen) of digestion so that the yang side (Stomach) can do its job properly.

Furthermore, in the morning try to eat something that has more liquid content while in the evening try to avoid overeating. This may seem to be contrary to the way Americans tend to eat. Please take these recommendations to heart as they reflect the feelings of my two friends Tu Hsin Wu and Wellington Xu.

Now we come to the topic of sexual relations (the "Big Desire" *dà yù* 大欲). It goes without saying that this is just as important to our health. I could talk to you about this for a month and still not be finished. There seems to be a difference in the attitudes towards sex held by Americans today and how the ancients of China thought about it. I, myself, have studied the morality of the ancients in great depth, and I understand the way our modern society views sexual relations as well. I find it difficult to find a middle ground between these two extremes. But I hope you will take what I have to say to heart in terms of your sexual behavior to avoid such extremes. Just as we were discussing eating and drinking habits, the same goes for sexual habits or what is called "The Great Desire" (*dà yù* 大欲). There are of course also lesser desires (*xiǎo yù* 小欲) such as money and fame. But what good is having a million dollars if I can't take it with me when I die? In former times, the Chinese used to have many wives; I still have friends who have several wives. This is called *yù*, "desire" or "lust." A man who has lots of money and power also wants to accumulate many women. But this is not the "Great Desire." "Great Desire" is that we have our basic needs met and can live on through future generations. If this "Great Desire" turns into lust, you will do something foolish like gorging yourself until you die. Likewise, if you have so many wives, won't you also deplete yourself? "Great Desire" means that if you don't eat you will die. Likewise, if none of us married and had children, wouldn't that be the end of our people? The reason we have sexual relations is to procreate, so that the seed is carried forward. The reason we eat is to live longer. The real purpose of money is not for wealth but to help you get your basic needs met: clothes to keep you warm, food to eat, a roof over your head. That is "Great Desire." The character for "desire" (*yù*) has many meanings.[310] Great Desire can easily change into lust and then you would say the reason to have sex is just for fun. My suggestion here is to try to find a middle way, to reduce the extreme ways of living that I am seeing here in the West. I don't expect you to be like the ancient sages, that would be too much. However, the classics describe different ages of sexual development: the calculations begin with a boy at 16 years old, and a girl at 14 years old.[311] This was considered the beginning of puberty. Modern humans have changed slightly since the time of the ancients, and now puberty begins earlier. For example, a child like this one sleeping here at eight years old loses his baby teeth. But remember that what we Chinese call eight years old, you here consider seven years old. And our seven is your six, that is when the teeth begin to change.[312] The development of the Kidney organ network (genitourinary system) is related to the maturation of the bones and teeth. At the age of sixteen (15 years in Western terms) for boys and fourteen (13 years) for girls, the Kidney network is considered to be mature. This is when the menstrual cycle begins for girls and boys produce sperm.[313] When this first begins, it can be used to make babies, but it mustn't be used foolishly. According to the classics, at the age of sixteen, a boy should have an orgasm only once a week. In a cycle of seven days, the sperm is then replenished. This implies that it takes seven days for each of the five organ networks to contribute to the making of healthy sperm.[314] The body is not a machine that can be used continuously. By the age of twenty-four years then it takes a two-week period to replenish the sperm, so one should only have an orgasm once every two weeks. This means that the creative abilities of the genitourinary system have slowed down by one week. By thirty-two years of age, it takes 3 weeks to replenish the sperm and by forty years of age, it takes 40 days. By fifty years old, it is no more. Doesn't that scare you? Now this idea was originally meant for someone to live to be 120 years old. The ancients felt that that was a natural span of human life. But nowadays, people are all taking out loans from the bank. If you go and borrow every day from the bank (of *jing*) there will come a day soon when you are bankrupt.

Here I am talking to you modern American youth, using these ancient Chinese terms to describe a completely different system of health. Don't you think that's a bit too much to ask of you? I am telling you this so that at least you can say you've heard it and be aware that such ideas exist.

What I am speaking about here are really these four characters that come from ancient human history.[315]

qīng xīn 清心
kuān yù 寬欲

Qīngxīn means to clear or settle one's Heart/mind. *Kuānyù* means to reduce or relax one's desires.

Humans are a type of animal. Though we consider ourselves more intelligent than monkeys, for example, all other animals—horses, sheep, cattle, dogs—have a mating season when they are in heat. It's only humans who are different. We humans can make a mess of things by doing whatever we want, whenever we want to. This is why I mention these four ancient characters. *Tàijí* practice is a great help in supporting this idea. When practicing *tàijí*, you concentrate on placing the mind in the *dāntián* 丹田, in your abdomen, and your spirit (*shén* 神) and breath (*qì* 氣) will settle there. If you practice *tàijí* in this way, each morning and evening, your mind will become very clear and your passions and desires will natural be reined in. Now when your desires for sex rise, beware that they do not become excessive. Do your best to reduce this and don't let your passions run away.

To finish then, we have six characters of health: drinking and eating , the big desire of sexual relations, and we also have waking and sleeping. I don't want to say too much more about this. Keep it simple. Don't oversleep, try to get 7-8 hours if you can. Why is this? Because a little less sleep makes the quality of sleep deeper and sweeter. It's easier to fall asleep this way. In Chinese this is called "Sweet Sleep."[316] For example, if last night I slept 8 ½ hours, then tonight when I go to bed, I may be tossing and turning, my mind traveling everywhere. Is this not troublesome? Also when you sleep, you should sleep on the right side, not the left. This is important! Your Heart is on the left side and so is the Stomach while the Liver is more on the right side than the left. The right side of the Lungs is also larger than the left, it has one additional section. So when you sleep on the right side, there is no fear of placing undue pressure on the Heart, Stomach or Lung. If you sleep on the left side, your Heart will be compressed and you will have bad dreams that will wake you up. Now sleeping on the right side takes some practice getting used to. It's easy to say "I'll sleep on the right side," but then you get tired of that position and turn over or turn over unconsciously during your sleep. Nevertheless, try to remind yourself to sleep more on the right side if you can.

So I will end with this: There is nothing better than *tàijí quán* 太極拳 for your health. Hearing me say this today, I hope you will be able to remember it in the future. I know a lot of you here have been patients of mine as well. And now because I am leaving, you may be wondering what you are going to do about staying healthy without me. Let me repeat once more: wake up at a set time each morning. Go to sleep at the same time each night. Eat and drink accordingly, as we have discussed. In this way, you will prevent disease. And if every day you develop these habits and practice *tàijí* to promote proper circulation of blood-*qì*, then you will be able to withstand any kind of drafts and colds and infections. And if you do develop the early signs of a problem, eat less and drink more and the illness won't become serious. This is better for you than any medicine. When something hurts, massage it over and over until it feels better. If you feel like a fever is beginning, eat less and drink more and it will be gone tomorrow. This is even better than the herbs I prescribe for you. I have been wanting to talk to you all about this and in a wink, a year has gone by. So today I have had a chance to speak with you, my friends and students and I am very happy to have had this opportunity. Although I don't have much longer to stay in America, at least we have had this chance to speak about good health. Of course, my number one hope is that you will continue to practice your *tàijí* faithfully in the morning and in the evening and don't forget, while you are practicing, to quiet your mind and place your breath in your abdomen.

That's enough for now. This is all you need. Have a nice year and I hope to see you all next year in good health.

Original Translation
Tam Gibbs and Ed Young December 16, 1975
(Edited by Stephen Cowan)

Appendix I Notes:

296 Among the many papers left to Ed Young from Professor Cheng was a translated copy of this lecture given in New York City that turns out to be his last lecture in the US before returning to Taiwan where he would later pass away.

---

297 Swami Bua (1889-2010) was a world renowned Yogi who taught Hatha Yoga in NYC during the 1960s and became a dear friend of Professor Cheng. There are a few photos of the two of them smiling together. In an article entitled *Hold It!* written by Anthony Hiss that appeared in the *New Yorker* October 29, 1973, it states: *"At the party thrown in honor of his upcoming trip to Taiwan (held at the Hwa Yaun Szechuan Inn, East Broadway) were Swami Bua, the Yogi, and Oscar Ichazo, the Bolivian founder of the Arica Institute. Cheng gave a speech (in Chinese) that emphasized the points of continuity in time, and balance. A documentary film about African bushmen, entitled "Bitter Melons," was shown before the party began."*

298 "Nurture life" Professor Cheng's discussion here concerns the concept of *yǎng shēng* 養生, a fundamental principle of Chinese culture and East Asian Medicine. The practice of fostering health and well-being in daily life focuses on nurturing body, mind and spirit in harmony with the natural circadian rhythms, and universal laws of *yīn-yáng*.

299 Zhou dynasty (*Zhōu dài* 周代) approximately 1046-256 BCE, considered the longest dynasty in China, was the time in which the major philosophies such as Confucianism and Daoism emerged.

300 *Jīn yè* 津液 (body secretion). See Chapter 13: The Mystery of Hormones.

301 In *yīn-yáng* theory, food nourishes the *yáng*, (meaning fuel for *qì*) and fluids nourish the *yīn*, meaning Blood. Qì and blood are a complementary pair.

302 As mentioned in *Sage Principles*, the blood (*yīn*) carries the qi (*yáng*) and the qi (*yáng*) moves the blood (*yīn*). Here, if the *qì* becomes depleted from excessive exercise, then eventually it will lead to stagnation of the blood (blood clots, high blood pressure, strokes etc.), causing serious health issues throughout the body.

303 "Swallowing the air" (*tūn tiān zhī qì* 吞天之氣) Literally: "swallowing the qì of heaven" is taken to mean breathing into the *dāntián* 丹田, part of Professor Cheng's famous quote to his students: "Swallow the Qì of Heaven, tap the strength of the ground and prolong life through softness." *Tūn* 吞 means "swallow," "absorb," or "take in." The character depicts an image of Heaven above a mouth.

304 *Dāntián* 丹田 (elixir field) see Chapter 9 .

305 This may be the same Dù Xīnwǔ 杜心武 mentioned in Smith, (1990). *Chinese Boxing, Masters and Methods,* p. 39, as one of the legendary Kungfu (*gōngfu* 功夫) martial arts masters.

---

306 Recent research has confirmed that mouthwashes suppress active ingredients in saliva important for our health. Saliva contains high concentrations of nitric oxide, a potent antioxidant which acts as a signaling molecule that regulates inflammation, vascular tone and insulin sensitivity, exerting a protective function in the lining of blood vessels and reducing inflammation markers. See Guo, et al. (2025), *Association of over-the-counter mouthwash use with markers of nitric oxide metabolism, inflammation, and endothelial function—a cross-sectional study.*

307 Spleen (*pí* 脾) from a strictly anatomic perspective, the pancreas may be considered as one aspect of the Spleen network's role in digestion. The pancreas sits directly next to and behind the Stomach / duodenum and is critical in activating digestion (see Chapter 13). However, it's important to note that, in five phase doctrine, the Spleen network serves many other roles in the body related to mental and physical functions beyond digestion.

308 In the medical classics, *Nèijīng* 《內經》 and *Nán Jīng* 《難經》, mind and body are never considered as two separate entities. Thus each physical organ has cognitive and spiritual powers associated with it. *Xìn* ("sincerity," "reliability," "trustworthiness") is said to be one of the spiritual powers associated with the Spleen.

309 "Kicks it into action" from a Western medical perspective, the exocrine and endocrine functions of the pancreas do in fact have a direct effect on stimulating the breakdown of food in the duodenum, which in East Asian medicine, is grouped as part of the Stomach *fǔ* 腑.

310 See Appendix III: *Etymological Glossary of Sage Principle Terms*, for a more detailed analysis of *yù* 欲, p. 191.

311 In traditional East Asian culture, a child is considered to be born at 1 year old. Therefore a boy of 16 years in East Asian calculations is actually 15 years old and a girl of 14 is actually 13 years old, according to our Western measurement.

312 Professor Cheng is quoting from the *Huángdì nèijīng* medical classics, *Sùwèn* Chapter 1 that refers to the so-called "cycle of sevens and eights": "*Qi Bo replies: "In a female, at the age of seven, The [first] teeth are substituted and the hair grows long. With two times seven, the heaven gui arrives, the controlling vessel is passable and the great thoroughfare vessel abounds [with qi]. The monthly affair moves down in due time and, hence, [a woman] may have children.* [...] *In a male, at the age of eight, the qi of the Kidneys is replete; his hair grows and the [initial] teeth are substituted. With two times eight, the qi of the Kidneys abounds; the heaven gui arrives and the essence qi flows away. Yin and yang find harmony. Hence, he can have children.* " Unschuld and Tessenow (2011) pp. 36-41.

Interestingly, since the 1960's there has been a slow downward shift in the age of menarche in girls that perhaps may relate to the rapid pace of our modern society, coupled with dietary changes towards more highly processed diet. See Ramraj, et al. (2021) *Study on Age of Menarche Between Generations and the Factors Associated With It.*

---

[313] *Jīngzǐ* 精子 (sperm) - For more on this see Chapter 13.

[314] In East Asian medical thinking, all five organ networks contribute to the creation of healthy sexual organ function. This includes many lifestyle practices that support healthy digestion, sleep-wake cycles and emotional balance.

[315] Though versions of this quote run through both the Confucian and Daoist classics, the closest direct quote we can find comes from the poem "Great Ming United" (*dàmíng yītǒng* 大明一統) found in the *Fēng xuān xuán pǐn* 風宣玄品 (1539) a Ming-dynasty *gǔqín* 古琴 tablature compiled by Zhū Hòujué 朱厚爝. This text contains technical essays and illustrations on *qín* 琴 playing and construction, followed by tablature for 101 melodies (34 with lyrics), many drawn from earlier musical traditions and sources. "*A clear Heart with few desires, adds years to lives full and strong.*" (*qīngxīn guǎ yù, yì shòu mí jiān jiàn zuò niàn kǔ, yù mín cóng qīng* 清心寡慾，益壽彌堅 踐祚念苦，欲民從輕。)

[316] *Hǎo mèng* 好梦 ("sweet sleep") is similar to saying "sweet dreams" in English.

Appendix II: Four Personal Recollections of Medical Treatment by Professor Cheng

Cheng Man-ch'ing as Doctor: A Recollection

Entering a cavernous loft with old oak floors and a wall of windows on one side, I filled an empty chair in the front row, seated directly opposite Cheng Man-ch'ing's hefty desk.

He was an imposing figure, with the feel of a stone Buddha due to the seeming density of his mass and the fact that he barely moved—no expressive gesticulation, no unnecessary movement of the hands, arms, or body of any kind. I had never witnessed a person with such deliberate stillness before. His manner was intent and measured, yet with a counterbalance of immense grace and a lightness of being. His presence was itself the commencement of a healing.

The protocol for being assessed by pulse diagnosis and issued a script for an herbal formula was to wait your turn. It was 1972. An adult man was listening to Cheng Man-ch'ing relay that the origin of his troubles occurred when he fell asleep beside a lake when he was seven years old, and this precipitated a chill to his Kidneys that had persisted.

I grew up as the daughter of a surgeon who trained in the early 1940s, when doctors were still taught to rely on their senses and before laboratory testing replaced clinical skills. But my dad was a dedicated materialist who believed that physical matter is the fundamental aspect of reality, and as such, would have been flummoxed by Cheng Man-ch'ing's diagnostic narrative including an incident at a lake that occurred decades prior contributing to a medical problem in present time.

It was my turn to sit in the chair perpendicular to Cheng Man-ch'ing's and lift my wrist onto the small pillow on his desk. With an economy of motion, he touched my arm with his fingers. When he attuned to me with his laser focus, he dropped out of character, letting his mouth open agape. His body language told me that although I looked like a robust 26-year-old, my pulse betrayed a weakness he was not expecting. I was impressed that without my telling him that I was unstable and fragile, he knew it, even if it surprised him.

He told me that because of a cascade of events, I had shortened my lifespan. He wrote out a prescription for Chinese herbs and told me to return when they ran out for a reassessment. At the far end of the studio, Ed Young was practicing a T'ai Chi Sword Form by himself. I walked past him, and out into the brisk New York air, feeling fortunate to have encountered a person seemingly from another time and place entirely.

Harriet Beinfield 2022
Co-Author with Efrem Korngold of *Between Heaven and Earth: A Guide to Chinese Medicine*

Medical Treatment of My Son by Professor Cheng

In early 1970 when my son, Denis, was 4 years old, a senior student of the Professor's told me about his teacher and how he could heal people. At that time, Denis was being seen by countless specialists at NY Medical College Mental Retardation Center and none of them were helping him. They had diagnosed him as "brain damaged," "autistic," "mentally retarded," and "emotionally disturbed." He was at that time attending a therapeutic preschool that had only two students and two certified special education teachers. They offered no help either.

Denis was banging his head violently, biting his hand, screaming and rocking. He could say several words but did not have any receptive language. He actually had no reciprocity at all. He seemed to be in his own tormented world. He could look but not see, hear but not listen. He was miserable and so was I.

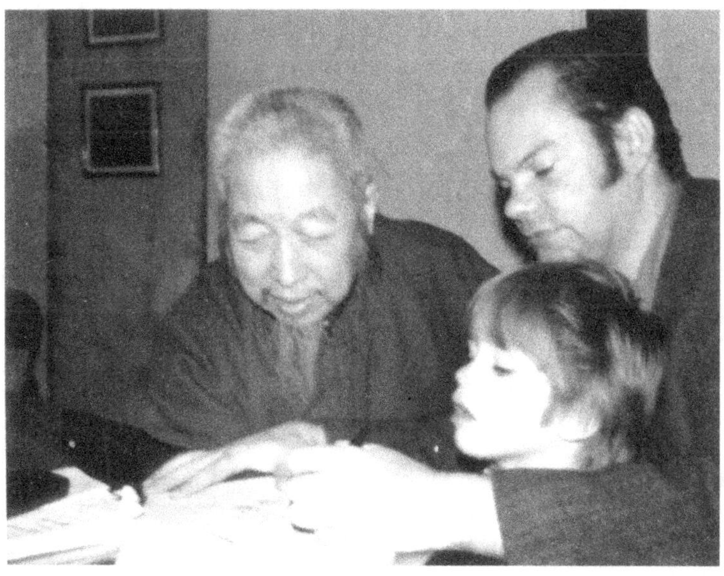

Professor Cheng with Tam Gibbs treating Denis

I liked the idea of seeing this doctor of Traditional Chinese Medicine and was hopeful as we walked up the stairs at 211 Canal Street. Denis stood on a bench and looked out the window onto Canal Street screeching at the lights from the cars and trucks. He was transfixed and over-stimulated as we waited for the Professor to arrive. After a bit, his translator (Tam Gibbs) came over and asked us to go to the desk where the Professor would examine Denis. Denis would not budge. He just would not move and I felt so awful to think that our chance for a healing was thwarted by this willful child. Well, as was consistent with how the Professor treated us for the next five years, he ascertained the situation and with compassion, came over to Denis. He felt his pulses and told me that Denis would get better and better as the years went by. He took Denis down from the bench by the window and held his hand as they walked over to the desk. Denis sat on Tam's lap and I listened. He said that Denis' blood was too hot when he was born and that his Liver was too strong. He said that Denis could not distinguish the foreground from the background and that his world was chaos. He could make me out because he was so used to me but did not really see others. He took out his brush and wrote down a prescription for the herbs I was to brew. I asked when we should come back, and he said we did not have to. My heart sank as I thought that this one-time visit could not really affect what Denis needed. He smiled with compassion and said that if I wanted to come back, I could come next week.

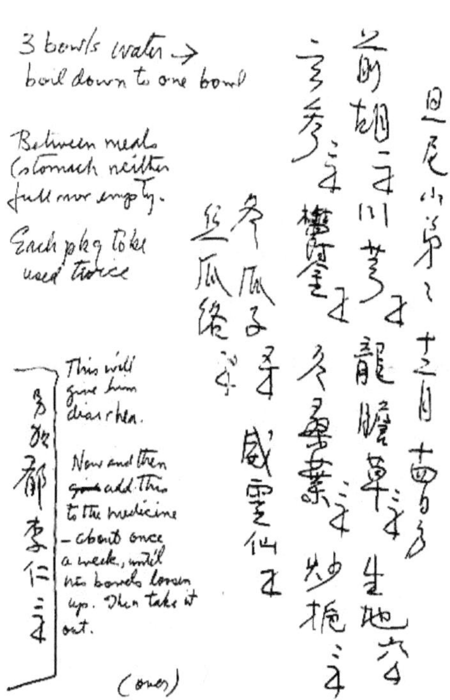

One of Professor Cheng's Prescriptions for Denis

So we began the treatment and came once or twice a week for the next five years. After the first few weeks Denis stopped banging his head. He just stopped! That, in itself, would have been enough of a healing but more came to us. After a few more weeks, Denis looked at a stranger on the street and said "hello!" He was able to see others. He began to pay attention to others, and I noticed that his motor skills were improving. He was soon able to get onto his rocking chair all by himself. Denis dragged one leg as he walked clumsily. His orthopedist had suggested that he wear two right shoes to try to correct how he walked with his feet placed outward like a duck. The Professor noted this and said that I should get Denis soft sneakers that would bend easily as he walked and that I should bend down and correctly position his feet once in a while, as the Professor's mother had done for him. Over time, his gait improved and he was much more like a normal little boy in his sneakers instead of his clunky orthopedic shoes.

Denis improved little by little and once early on, when I realized the Professor was going on a trip to Taiwan, my heart sank. I worried that our chance for healing would end. The Professor ascertained my feelings and told me that if my need was great enough, no distance, not even 8,000 miles, could cause us to be separated. I felt reassured and whenever he would go to Taiwan, I would stay in touch with him with my heart by way of Tam and he would come to the rescue with a prescription of herbs sent from Taiwan with careful instructions as needed.

One day, the Professor noted by way of Denis' pulses, that he had been wetting himself. He was concerned about this and told me there was a treatment. I was to find fertilized chicken eggs and as soon as one hatched I was to twist its neck, take off the feathers and beak and cook it for Denis to eat in a sandwich. He told me not to let Denis see this and not to let him know what he was eating. After several chick treatments, we returned to the Professor, who said he was getting better but that I had to do one more series of treatments. I told him that I could not do this again. It had taken all my strength and I just could not do it. The Professor was quite firm on this and said I had no choice. He said that Denis would grow up wetting himself if I did not do it again. Well, I did and it worked!

The Professor always welcomed us to see him at the Taichi studio at 211 Canal Street and 87 Bowery. No matter what fuss Denis made, we were always welcome. He would send Tam over to get us sometimes as I was embarrassedly packing up to leave abruptly. He would watch and give his attention to the many drawings Ed or Tam would do for Denis as he was seen for his visit. I recall one time when Denis grabbed the Professor's papers and would not let go. I tugged and tugged to get them and the Professor smiled and said not to pull them and let him have them and the Professor kept giving him papers, yielding until finally Denis just let go.

Denis' life has had challenges but the healing that occurred in those years has helped him learn to relate to others, care about others, and find joy in life. He shows reverence whenever the Professor's name is mentioned. He has reciprocity in language and in life. He is not at all in his own world. He joined the world and is able to garnish what he needs from the universe. He has been blessed.

As you can see in the photo from 2018, Denis has his humanity.

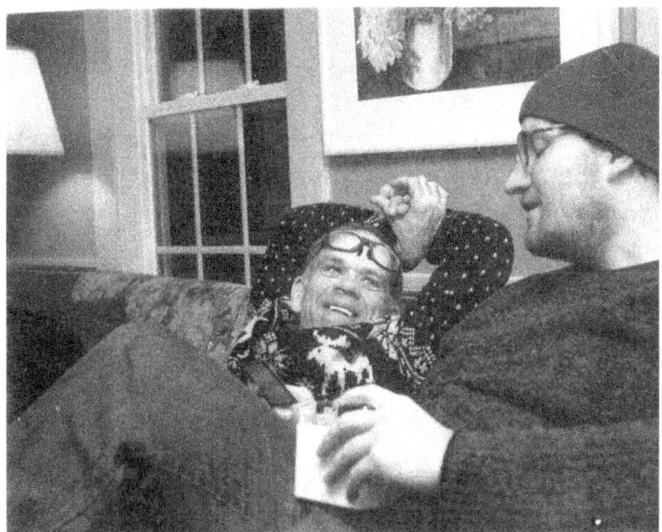

Denis (left) conversing with a friend

Prepared for Ed Young by Barbara Penna Goldsmith
February 7, 2020
Ed has permission to use and edit any of this material as he sees fit.

Fatigue and Flank Pain in a Young Mother

In early 1970, I began treatment with Professor Cheng. I was experiencing some fatigue and pain in my left side. The Professor felt my pulses and told me that my Kidney was weak. I asked him if that was what caused my son to be born so unwell. He said "influenced but did not cause!" I began taking the herbal brew he prescribed and slowly felt better. After a few treatments he asked me about my menstrual cycle. I told him that my periods came about every 33-34 days and that my family doctor told me that that was normal for me. He shook his head and said that the doctor was wrong and that the cycle of menstruation was related to the moon cycle and should be (ideally) every 28 days. He asked me to show him the color of the blood in my flow as he offered several small pillows with variations of the color red. When I selected the pale red color, he shook his head and said that that was not good and showed me the rich color that it should be. After several months taking the herbal brew, which the Professor tweaked each week as he examined my pulses, my period was straightened out and came every 28 days and was the correct color. This lasted for over two decades. I felt stronger and stronger and believe that the Professor helped me to be strong enough to accept the challenges of having a sick child who was quite vulnerable and needed my unconditional love and care as well as his sister.

Over the five years that the Professor uncannily questioned me, he offered me comments that opened my thinking to the possibility that the spirit was in the flesh, that mind and body were one, and that hope was available. This has proven to be quite significant in my life. Prior to 1970 I was not at all open to any of these concepts and felt quite estranged and a bit hopeless.

A year or so after the the Professor passed, I was taking a class at the Center for Asian studies at St. John's University and Tam Gibbs happened to be in my class. At Tam's suggestion and encouragement, we visited Madame Cheng twice at her home in Queens on Hillside Avenue. While we were there, some of her family members came by, as it was Lunar New Year. I was surprised to find that they knew me and Denis (my son). It was touching that this would have been the case since my whole family, of course, knew of Professor Cheng. It was quite special to spend time with Madame Cheng as she spoke with me of how the lotus has roots down in the muddy waters and when flowering, rises up towards the heavens. She compared this to the relationship of Earth, Man and Heaven. That day in our class at St. Johns, Tam and the teacher of the class talked about the significance of incense and how to use it and hold it and raise it up three times to connect with the spirit of one who has passed. I was therefore prepared and able to go over to the alter that was set up in Madame Cheng's home for the Professor and use the incense as I honored the good and learned friend who helped me so much.

Prepared for Ed Young by Barbara Penna Goldsmith
February 7, 2020
Ed has permission to use and edit any of this material as he sees fit.

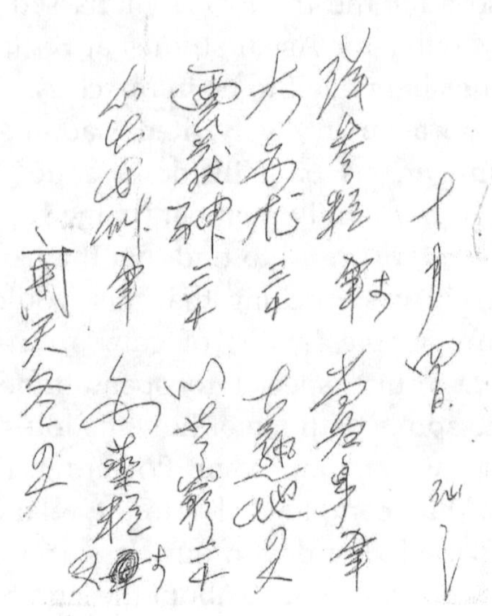

慶餘堂參藥號有限公司
CHING YUE TARNG CHINESE MEDICINE & GINSENG CO., LTD.
NO. 34, SECTION 2, SHIN YI ROAD
TAIPEI, TAIWAN

TELEPHONE:
28008

CERTICATE OF ORIGIN

Issued at: Taipei, Taiwan
Republic of China
Date: August 14, 1972

This is to certify that undermentioned commodity, mailed from Taipei on August 14, 1972 was manufactured by Ching Yue Tarng Chinese Medicine & Ginseng Co., Ltd. consigned to Mrs Barbara Penna that is of Taiwan origin:

Buyer: Mrs Barbara Penna, 148-31, 60 Ave. Flushing 11355, New York, USA.
Comodity: Stomachic Pill
Quantity: 270 Gm.
Effposition: Indigestion, Anorexia
Composition: Cassia oddidentalis
Areca catechu Linn
Dioscorea Japonica, Thunb
Coix Lachryma Jobi (Chinese Medicine Herb)
Manufacturer: Ching Yue Tarng Chinese Medicine & Ginseng Co., Ltd.
Supplier: Ching Yue Tarng Chinese Medicine & Ginseng Co., Ltd.
Packing: Paper Box with P. E. Bag.

Ching Yue Tarng Chinese Medicine & Ginseng Co., Ltd.

James Kuo
Sales Manager

JK/sp

Sample prescription by Professor Cheng written for Barbara with Translation from Taipei Pharmacy.

Treated by Professor

I ended up seeing Professor medically many times, because the first time was the convincer. Following Tam's advice, I had gone in for an introductory check up. Professor read my pulses then said (I don't remember whether the translator was Ed or Tam), "You've got a cold around your heart."

About three years before starting my Taichi study, I had come down with a painful case of pericarditis, an inflammation of the heart lining. The thing had me in bed for months until I finally "returned to health." However, in the following few years I always had the feeling – that would come when I was overly tired – well, it felt like "a cold around my heart."

Professor gave me a prescription which was my first experience of that terrible tasting tea, "the very soul of bitterness." I don't remember how long the treatment lasted, not long though longer than the subsequent times I was treated by him. By the end the illness really was gone, never to return. Which always happened, whenever I consulted him medically.

Wolfe Lowenthal
One of Professor Cheng's early students in NYC
Founder of Long River Taichi and author of
There Are No Secrets, Gateway to the Miraculous, & Like a Long River

Appendix III: *Etymological Glossary of Sage Principle Terms*

Ed Young discovered Chinese seal characters from Cheng Man-ch'ing and fell in love with them for what they evoked in him. Prior to that discovery, he hadn't really thought about the characters of his native Chinese language as pictures. Being an artist, he found whole worlds in each character he met as they came alive in their original oracle bone, bronze and seal forms, allowing the ancients to speak in the present. He passed that study/play on to me thirty years ago, and I am deeply grateful for that gift, for like the "old friends" Ed said these characters would become to me, their true meanings change with the context of each meeting, showing me something about who and how I am at a particular moment of time.

It is our hope that these characters will evoke something unique to you as you chew on them and digest them. As Zhuāngzǐ says of "goblet words" (*zhīyán* 卮言),[317] these characters are filled with meanings for you, only to be emptied out, once swallowed and ready to fill again with different meanings the next time you taste them.

Stephen Cowan 2026[318]

Bāguà 八卦 the eight divinatory trigrams of the *Yìjīng* 《易精》(*Book of Changes)*

Bā 八 "eight, all around"

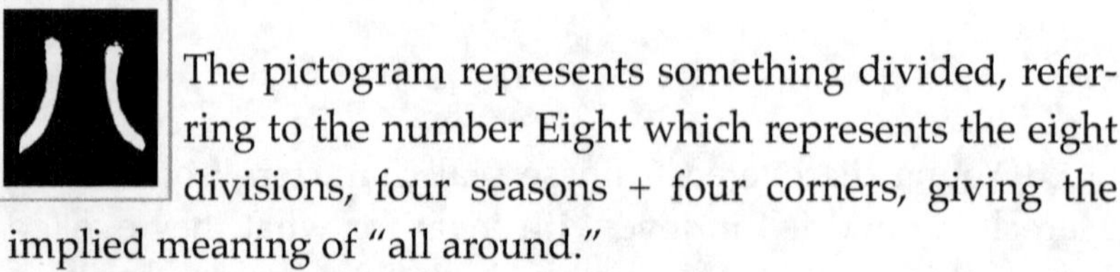

The pictogram represents something divided, referring to the number Eight which represents the eight divisions, four seasons + four corners, giving the implied meaning of "all around."

Guà 卦 "trigram"

On the right this ancient ideogram is thought to represent a cracked bone or turtle shell used in divination. On the left may be a representation of the pattern left after heating the turtle shell that gives a hexagram.

Biàntōng 變通 "change and continuity, or "flux and flow," meaning "free flowing change, pragmatic; flexible; to act differently in different situations; to accommodate to circumstances." This important term defines the constancy of change. It appears many times throughout the *Yìjīng* 《易精》*(Book of Changes).*

Biàn 變 "to change, transform, transition"

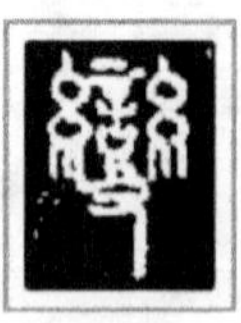

The image of a mouth speaking *yán* 言 is placed between two strands of twisted silk, *luán* 䜌 which by itself represents the entanglements of speech, meaning confusion or argument. Below this is a hand holding a baton or stick, (*pū* 攴) which represents someone taking control, like a conductor of an orchestra. Together the ideogram *Biàn* implies the active role of moving through confusion of change.

***Tōng* 通:** "to go, move, to flow unobstructed, to communicate, to lead to, to reach, to understand thoroughly, to let through, to be fluent."

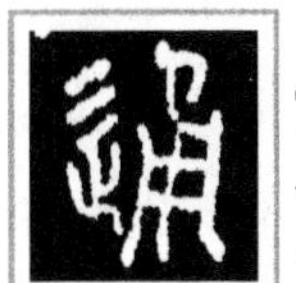

The image depicts a foot moving on the left of what is thought to be a budding plant or a bell. *Tōng* is an important term in East Asian medicine, representing health through the free flowing communication within the vessels and between the organs as well as between people, meaning to communicate verbally in a coherent way.

***Dāntián* 丹田**: the so-called "elixir field" or "cinnabar field" in Daoist cultivation located in the abdomen. See Chapter 9.

***Dān* 丹:** "cinnabar, red mineral, elixir."

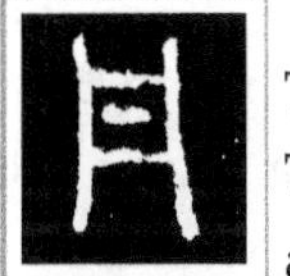

This is said to be a pictogram of a well or a mine. The central dot or line is used to accent the point at which the precious substance (elixir) is found. The Daoists used this concept of the *dān* to represent the alchemist's crucible with cinnabar in it.

Tián 田 "a cultivated field"

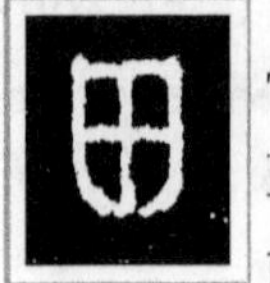

This image is said to represent a four-square field. In ancient times farmland was divided into four plots, all sharing a central well. In *dāntián*, this represents the field of internal cultivation of the elixir.

Dào 道"road, path, method, Way, process."

The ideogram contains on the left an image of a foot moving along a path next to a head perhaps with hair or feathers implying "a chief." One might say *Dào* is the process of "*heading* down the road."

Dū 督 "to oversee, supervise"

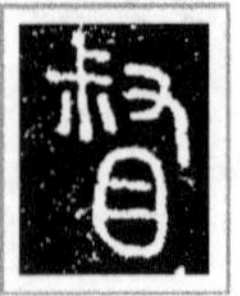

The ideogram contains a combined image of a plant with a hand, meaning "uncle or advisor," below which is the image of an eye. Taken together the implied meaning is to oversee or supervise. In East Asian medicine, *dū* refers to the channel running along the spine from the sacrum up to the head and is often referred to as the "Governor Vessel" (*dū mài* 督脈). It is considered *yang* relative to the "Conception Vessel" (*rèn mài* 任脈) (see below). See Chapter 8 and 13.

Duì 兌 "to exchange, pleasure, laughing, to gather." It is one of the eight *bāguà* 八trigrams ☱ with inferred meaning "stream, swamp, marsh, pond."

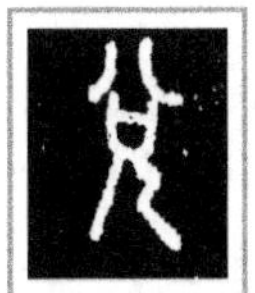

The image is said to depict an open smiling mouth with arms and legs dancing. This old image may simply be a pictorial representation of the trigram ☱ (a *yīn* line at the surface of two dancing *yáng* lines). It may also be an image representing an opening (or mouth) where water pours in. There is a quality of pleasure in this image, like the sound of a laughing stream in Springtime. Among the eight trigrams *bāguà* 八 it symbolizes the action/principle of gathering streams in a marsh or pond.

Fēng 風 "wind, airs, manners, atmosphere" see also association with trigram *xùn* 巽 [☴] (see character translation below).

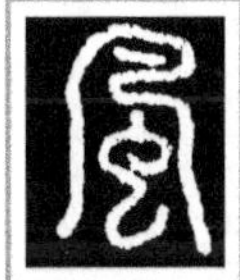

The image of atmospheric currents moving and swirling around a little insect. In East Asian culture, it was believed that insects were born on the wind. In fact they are borne on the wind.

Hùndùn **混沌:** "primordial chaos"

Hùn **混:** "to mix, mingle, blend, confused, muddy."

The image of water appears to the left of an image of the sun under which are two people, meaning a multitude or different kinds mingling.

Dùn 沌: "murky, confused, turbid, unclear, chaotic." *Dùn* also has the implied meaning of "spontaneity" or "innocence of a baby."

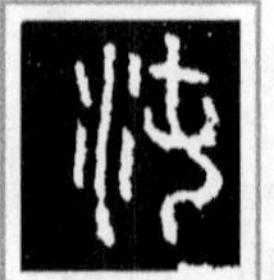

The image of water appears to the left of a plant emerging beneath the ground. The combined term *hùndùn* 混沌 in Chinese mythology represents the primal or primordial chaos or the formless mass that exists before the differentiation into *yīn-yáng* (for more on *hùndùn* see the story in *Zhuāngzǐ* 莊子 Chapter 7).

Gèn 艮: "obstinate, blunt, solid," one of the Eight Trigrams *bāguà* 八卦, symbolizing mountain ☶.

The image of a person turning around to look directly in the eye at someone or something. It corresponds to the austere action/principle of mountain stillness, solitude, solitary, solid: one *yáng* line above two *yīn* lines indicating a solid base.

Húnpò 魂魄: "soul-spirits"

Hún 魂: "ethereal soul-spirit"

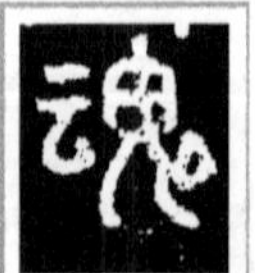

The image of a cloud appears to the left of a ghost/spirit (*guǐ* 鬼). In Chinese medical texts, *Hún* is referred to as the "ethereal soul" associated with the Wood phase and Liver organ network and is that aspect of our soul that flies off during dreams and when we lose consciousness or die (see Chapter 4).

***Pò* 魄:** "corporeal soul/spirit"

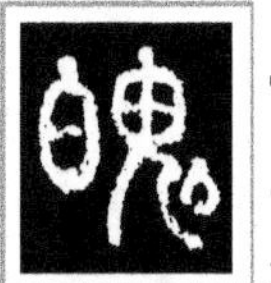

The image on the left depicts the sun with a dot above it, implied meaning "white" or "clear." This is placed next to an image of a ghost/spirit (*guǐ* 鬼) on the right. In East Asian medicine, *Pò* is associated with the Metal phase and Lung organ network and is considered the part of our soul-spirit that is left as white bones after we die (see Chapter 4).

***Jí* 極:** "extreme, extremely, highest, topmost, farthest, the utmost pole, to reach, arrive at"

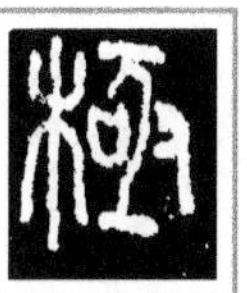

The image of a tree, implied meaning "natural," is placed to the left of a person flanked by a mouth and hand, all wedged between two horizontal lines representing the heavens and earth. The hand and mouth are thought to represent the two evolutionary skills (language and tool making) we humans developed to survive. In *tàijí* 太極, *tài* 太 means "vast or greatest" when coupled with *jí* it's often translated as "the great ultimate" or "greatest polarity," referring to the *yīn-yáng* symbol of interconnected polarities (*Taiji tu*) which represents the transformation of things as they move beyond their extreme. Note: The East Asian concept of "*Polarity*" contrasts with the Western duality of "*Dichotomy,*" as Roger Ames notes: "*The Sage recognizes and is skilled at facilitating harmony not as a fixed point but as the ever-changing shifting polarity along the continuum*"[319]

***Jīng* 精:** "essence, semen, vitality"

The image of a rice kernel (*mǐ* 米) on the left is placed next to the character *qīng* 青, "green" which corresponds to "the color of the East." In the correlative cosmology, Wood generates Fire, and the character incorporates *shēng* 生, "to generate" above *dān* 丹, "cinnabar/ elixir," which symbolically evokes the arousal and emergence of life. Together, *jīng* refers to the smallest component essential for life. See *jīngshén* 精神 ("essence-spirit") the fundamental mind-body relationship in East Asian medicine.

***Jīng* 經:** "a channel, to pass through, to undergo, to endure, a classic scripture that has been passed down through the ages."

The ideogram contains a string of twined silk to the left of an underground stream or aquifer. This ideogram has multiple meanings: in East Asian medicine, it refers to the acupuncture channels that carry blood and *qì* throughout the body. *Jīng* is also used to refer to a classic book, a sacred scripture or a woven textile that has been passed down through the ages such as *Dàodé jīng* 《道德經》*(the Classic of the Way and its Power)* or *Nèijīng* 《內經》 (*the Internal Medicine Classic*).

Jīnyè 津液: "saliva and body fluids"

Jīn 津: "saliva, to ferry, to ford a stream"

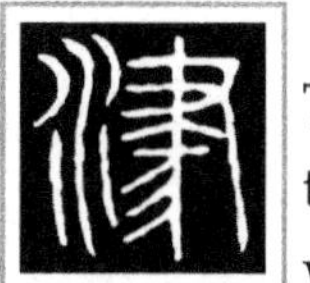

The water radical, indicating fluid, is placed next to an image of a hand holding a pole, as in one who fords a stream. In Chapter 13, Professor Cheng describes *jīn* as having a more *yáng* nature relative to *yè* (see description below).

Yè 液: "fluid, sap, juice, liquid"

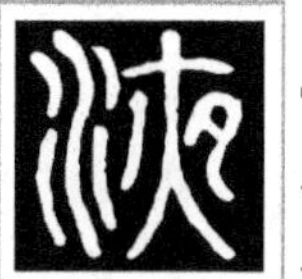

The water radical indicating fluid is placed next to a person holding the moon under the armpit, meaning dark night, possibly a reference to sweaty armpits or other dark places where bodily fluids accumulate. This moon radical gives *yè* a more *yīn* nature relative to *jīn* and is often associated with digestive secretions.

Jūn 君: "sovereign, chief, prince"

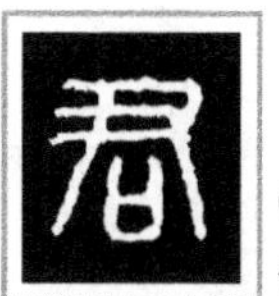

The image shows a mouth under a hand holding a cane, implying one who is cultivated and has mastered language or an elder who speaks wisely based on experience. *Jūnzi* 君子 is the Confucian ideal of a gentleman, an exemplary person of refined and mature manner. For the use of *zǐ* 子 (child, master, seed) see description below. From a *tàijí* perspective, the *yīn-yáng* aspects of *jūnzǐ* can be seen to represent both the *yáng*: mastery/power, refinement and the *zǐ*: softness, gentleness (gentility) of the cultivated "highly evolved" person.

***Kǎn* 坎:** "to sink, a pit, whirlpool, threshold, hole, snare; trap," one of the Eight Trigrams *bāguà* 八卦, symbolizing water ☵ (*kǎn* 坎)

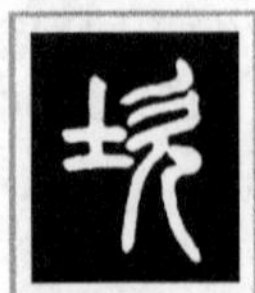

The image of soil next to a person exhaling, it relates to the action/principle of water carving the earth (like Ed's beloved Hudson river). Trigram ☵ *yáng* current running through the middle of *yīn*.

***Kē* 剋:** "to overcome or cut down"

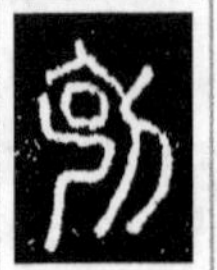

The image on the left is a person shouldering a heavy weight. On the right is a carving knife. In East Asian medicine, *Kē* refers to the inter-controlling forces within the five phases that counterbalance *shēng* 生 (see below).

***Kè* 客:** "guest, traveler, visitor, customer."

Within the image of a shelter, a person travels a path (two legs with a line running through it) below which is the image of a mouth. This ideogram represents a traveler stopping for shelter and food. When paired with *qì* 氣 (air, breath, atmosphere, action), *Kèqì* 客氣 means "courtesy, modesty, politeness," an important concept in Confucian practice.

***Kūn* 坤:** "receiving," one of the Eight Trigrams (*bāguà* 八卦), symbolizing "Earth" ☷ three *yīn* lines.

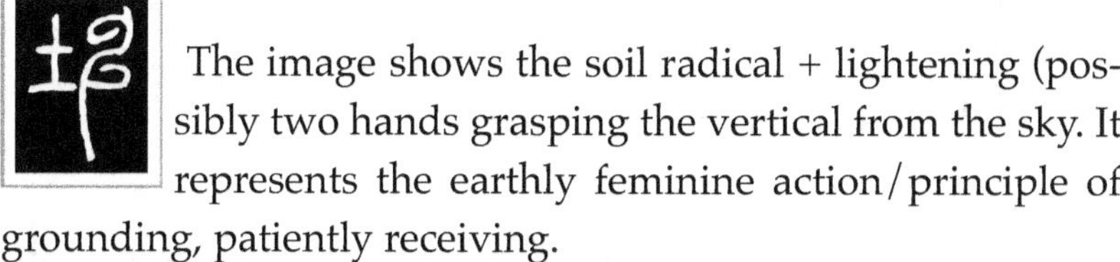

The image shows the soil radical + lightening (possibly two hands grasping the vertical from the sky. It represents the earthly feminine action/principle of grounding, patiently receiving.

***Lǎozǐ* 老子:** "old sage." It is the name of the legendary composer of the *Dàodé jīng* 《道德经》 during the Warring States period of the Zhou Dynasty (475-221 BCE).

***Lǎo* 老:** "old, wise"

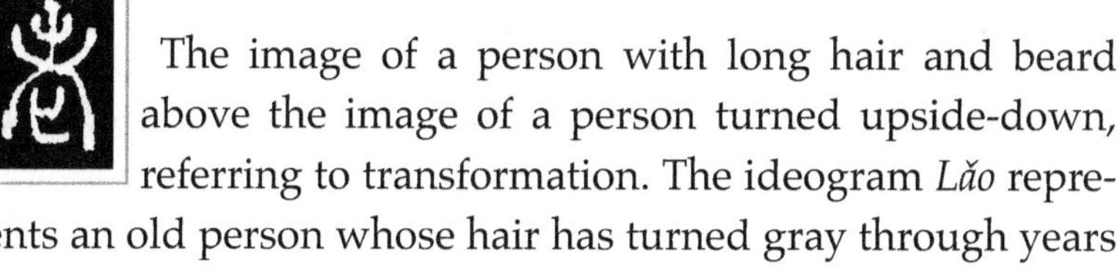

The image of a person with long hair and beard above the image of a person turned upside-down, referring to transformation. The ideogram *Lǎo* represents an old person whose hair has turned gray through years of experience.

***Zǐ* 子 (Tzu):** "child, seed, master"

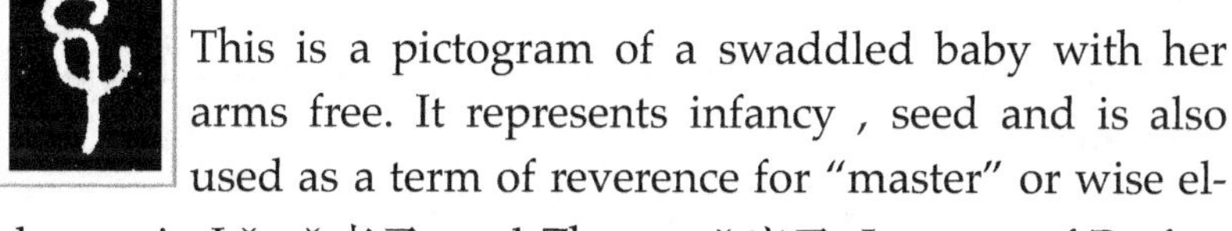

This is a pictogram of a swaddled baby with her arms free. It represents infancy , seed and is also used as a term of reverence for "master" or wise elders as in Lǎozǐ 老子, and Zhuāngzǐ 庄子. In some of Professor's posthumous texts, Cheng Man-ch'ing is referred to as Cheng-Tzu, (Zheng-zi), Master Cheng.

***Léi* 雷:** "thunder"

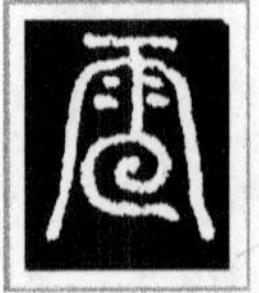

The image above of rain coming from the clouds onto the field below, creating a whirlwind. See related term *zhèn* 振 below.

***Lí* 離:** "to fly off, depart, leave, separate, distant." One of the Eight Trigrams (*bāguà* 八卦), symbolizing Fire ☲.

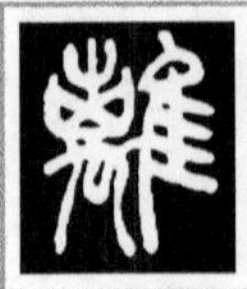

The image of a yak and a bird, said to be a mythological flying beast, perhaps a phoenix, that flies off high into the sky. It represents the action/principle of fire rising up, represented by ☲ a *yīn* in the middle of *yáng*.

***Liangyi* 兩儀** "two Modes, two forms, two appearances." According to Professor Cheng, the two modes are the *yīn-yáng* aspects of all things in nature expressed in trigrams *Qián* ☰ and *Kūn* ☷ which serve as the progenitors for the six "children" trigrams (see Chapter 3). Another interpretation of the Two Modes (*liangyi*) is one *yáng* straight line (—) and one *yīn* broken line (– –) which, in turn, generate the four double-lined images (*sì xiàng* 四象), which, in turn, generate the eight trigrams (see below).

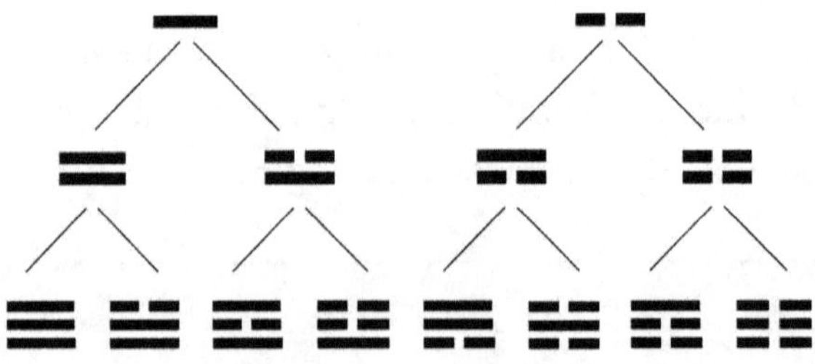

***Liǎng* 兩:** "two, a couple, a pair"

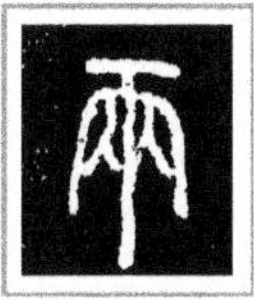

This image is said to show a balance or scale with two equal weights.

***Yí* 儀:** "apparatus, appearance, mode, instrument, rites,"

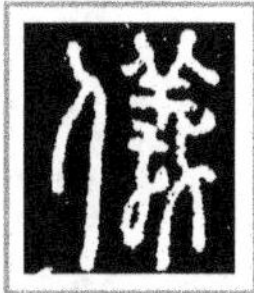

The image of a person facing to the left of *Yì* 義 meaning righteous (see below.)

***Líng* 靈:** "spirited, lively, clever, quick, alert, efficacious, effective."

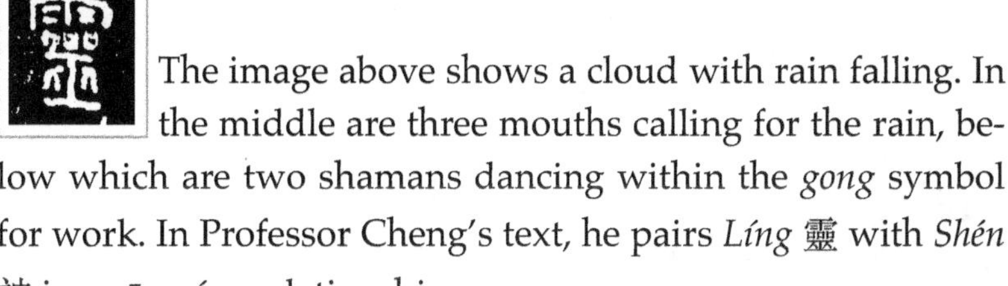

The image above shows a cloud with rain falling. In the middle are three mouths calling for the rain, below which are two shamans dancing within the *gong* symbol for work. In Professor Cheng's text, he pairs *Líng* 靈 with *Shén* 神 in a *yīn-yáng* relationship.

***Mài* 脈 (mo):** "arteries, veins, vessels, pulse, veins in a leaf."

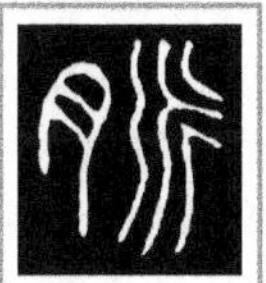

The image shows the "flesh" radical on the left, implying this is a bodily function. On the right is the image of flowing water in a channel.

Mìng 命: *"life, destiny, fate, decree"*

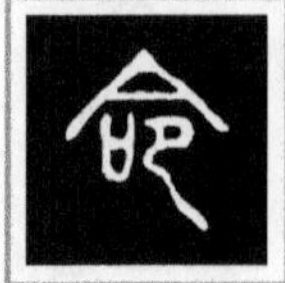

The image of a triangle above, said to be a symbol of unity below which is a mouth and a scepter, implied meaning a decree, command or mission. When *mìng* 命 is paired with *mén* 門 *(gate), mìng mén* 命門 means "gate of life" or "gate of destiny." This energetic center is located at the lower border of the second lumbar vertebrae (between the Kidneys, behind the *dāntián* 丹田). The *mìng mén* acupoint *Dū* 4 on the back is located directly across from *qì hǎi* 氣海, "the Sea of Qì" point (*Rèn* 6) on the front of the body and together give access to the *dāntián*. Activation of *Dū* 4 is said to improve Kidney/adrenal function, and promote *jīngqì* circulation, accessing the so-called original *qì* (*yuánqì* 元氣).

***Qì* (ch'i) 氣:** "animating vital force of life, breath."

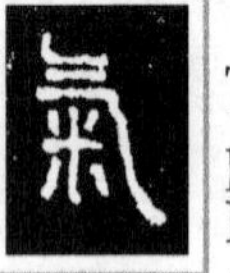

This ideogram shows a rice kernel with a cooking pot lid from which steam is rising. The term used in East Asian medicine refers to the vital animating force of life, literally the "breath of life." In the Professor's text, (Chapter 3) he describes three forms of *qì*: *tiānqì* 天氣, (heavenly atmospheric *qì*, the air we breathe), *xuèqì* 血氣 (the *qì* that moves blood) and *jīngqì* 精氣 (congenital *qì* given to use from our parents.) In East Asian medicine, *qì* represents the activation of all metabolic functions of the body/mind and is differentiated from the Daoist symbol *qì* 炁 that represents the warming effect of primordial *qì* in cultivation practice (see below).

***Qì* 炁:** "esoteric or primordial warming breath"

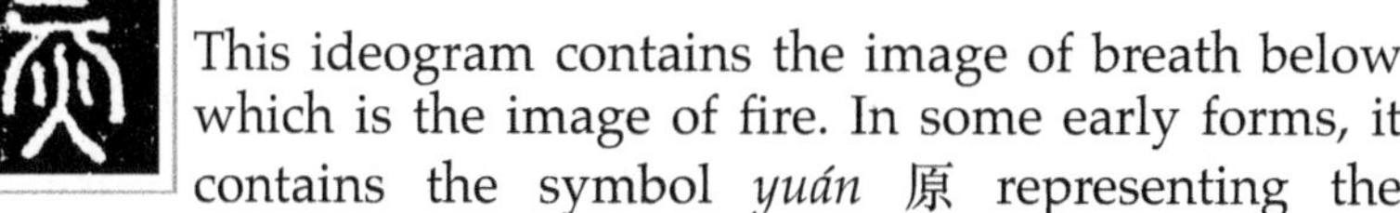

This ideogram contains the image of breath below which is the image of fire. In some early forms, it contains the symbol *yuán* 原 representing the source. *Qì* 炁 is an ancient Daoist symbol representing the warming breath used in cultivation practices. Professor Cheng uses *qì* 炁 to differentiate this primordial energy of cultivation from metabolic *qì* 氣 (see above). Though we have no easy translation for this term, it might be called "esoteric breath."

***Qián* 乾:** "the heavens, sunrise, vapors rising, drying," one of the Eight Trigrams (*bāguà* 八卦,) symbolizing the heavens ≡.

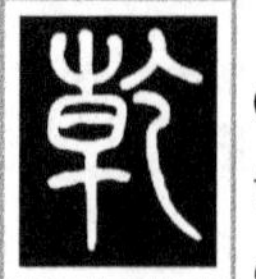

On the left, a sun rising through trees, symbolizing the East, on the right is an image of vapors rising at dawn. The implied meaning: the heavenly generative masculine *yáng* principle penetrating, and fertilizing (three *yáng* lines ≡). It represents the warming action/principle of the sun/sky.

***Qū Tū* 曲凸:** "bending and protruding"

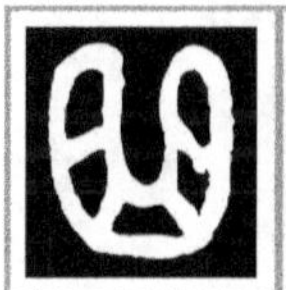
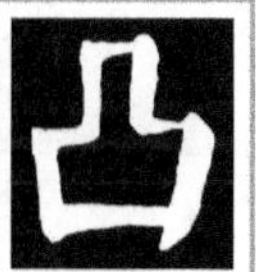

Qū image of a basket using bent bamboo. *Tū* image of a kind of puzzle piece or tongue and groove. See pp. 97-98 and footnotes 227 & 228 in reference to the body's proper position when sitting.

Rèn 任: "to bear, duty, responsibility, to rely upon."

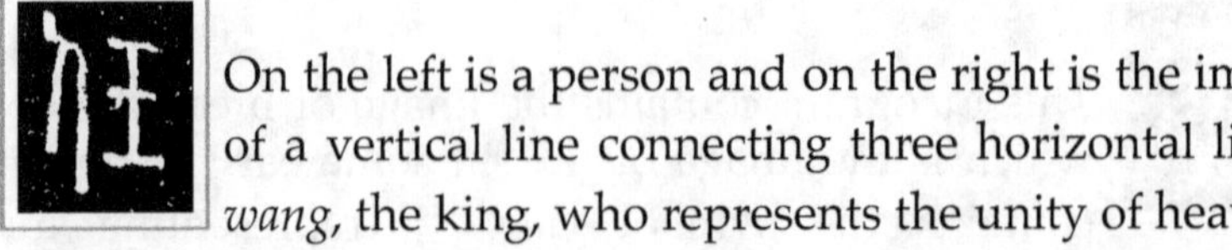

On the left is a person and on the right is the image of a vertical line connecting three horizontal lines, *wang*, the king, who represents the unity of heaven-earth-human. In East Asian medicine, *Rèn* refers to the front midline channel and is often translated as the "conception vessel" as it relates to nurturing life (Heart, womb, breasts etc.) *Rèn* is considered *yin* relative to the *Du*-back channel (see above).

Rén 仁: "humaneness, benevolence, kindness, universal love"

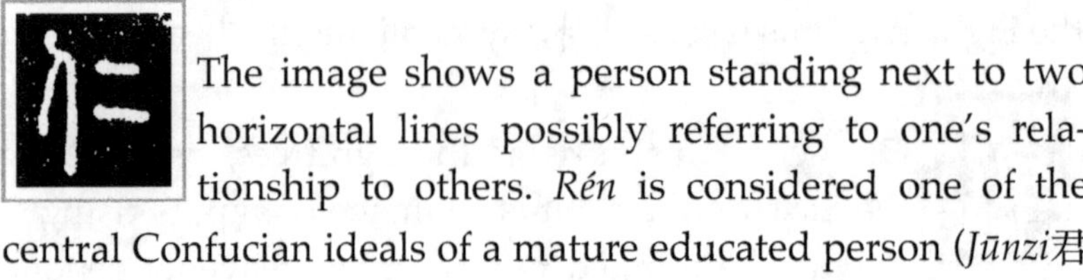

The image shows a person standing next to two horizontal lines possibly referring to one's relationship to others. *Rén* is considered one of the central Confucian ideals of a mature educated person (*Jūnzi*君子.)

Shān 山: "mountain"

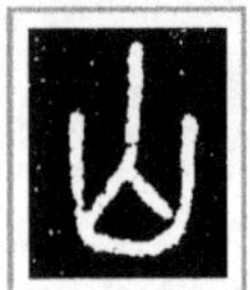

The image of a mountain peak flanked by two smaller peaks. It corresponds to the trigram *Gèn* 艮 ☶ (see above).

Shén 神: "divine spirit, awareness, consciousness, charisma."

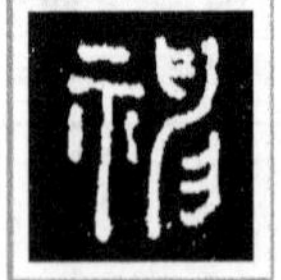

The image on the left shows the heavens (two horizontal lines) with three vertical lines coming down from them, representing the lights of the heavens, i.e. the sun, moon and stars. By itself this means "to reveal." On the right is an image of two hands grasping a rope (or possibly lightning). Together *Shén* gives the meaning of grasping divine light of spiritual awareness.

Shēng 生: "birth, life, living, to give rise to"

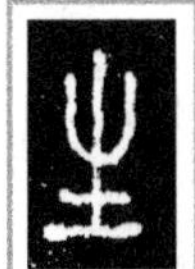

This is a pictogram of a plant emerging from the ground. In East Asian medicine, *Shēng* refers to the nourishing cycle of the five phases that counterbalances *Ke* (see above).

Shèng 聖: "saint, holy, wise sage"

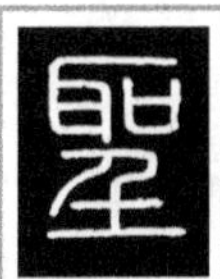

The ideogram depicts a person bowing below the ear and mouth – implied meaning: a wise person who listens before speaking.

Shí 實: "full, solid, true, real, honest, ripe"

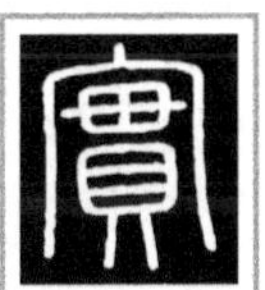

The image of a string of shells under a roof, implied meaning of fullness or richness (shells were a kind of money in ancient China.) In East Asian medicine, *Shí* - fullness makes a couple with *Xū* emptiness (see below).

Wěiguān gǔ 尾閲骨: "tailbone gate."

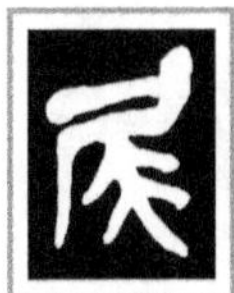 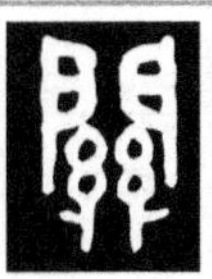 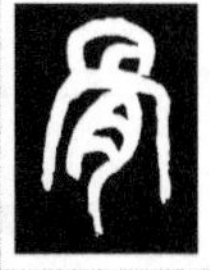

Wěi ideogram shows a tail coming from the seat of a crouching figure. *Guān* image of an open gate. *Gǔ* the image is thought to be that of a skeleton meaning "bone." *Wěiguān gǔ* is considered one of the three important "gates" in the Daoist meditative practice of the microcosmic orbit (see Chapter 13).

***Xiàng* 象**: "shape, form, appearance, likeness (a portrait), image, snapshot, phenomenon, the outward appearance or expression of anything, especially weather."

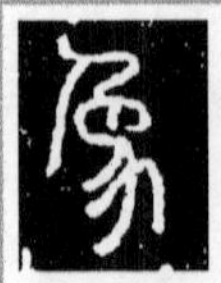

The image of an elephant may refer to the ivory used to carve a likeness or the idea of something very big that can be seen.

***Xīn* 心**: " Heart/mind", "core"

Said to be a pictogram of the Heart chambers, or possibly a picture of a flower blooming. In East Asian philosophy, the Heart and mind are considered as one central aspect of human body/mind unity of consciousness, the so called "distributed mind."

***Xìng* 性**: "one's nature, character, type"

On the left is the image for Heart/mind and on the right is the image of a plant emerging from the ground (*shēng* 生) which is the symbol for birth and life. *Xìng* is therefore the Heart/mind we are born with, our original nature.

***Xū* 虛:** "empty, barren, void"

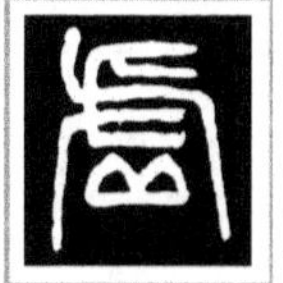

The image is of a tiger above two mountains, implied meaning: the empty barren places where tigers roam. In East Asian medicine, empty *Xū* is contrasted with fullness *Shí* (see above).

***Xué* 學:** "learning or teaching"

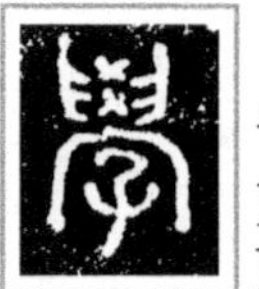

Above is an image of two hands reaching down, passing down information, literally demonstrating how to write an "x" with a second "x" being copied. Below is a shelter in which we see a child. See Chapter 1: "Sage Teachings" (*zhé xué* 哲學).

***Xùn* 巽:** "to obey, to submit, mild, modest." It is one of the Eight Trigrams (*bāguà* 八卦) symbolizing Wind ☴

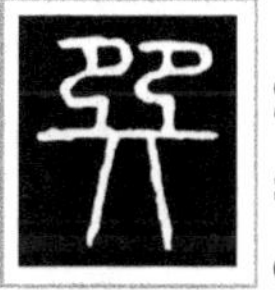

Some sources say it is an image of two kneeling servants over a table, implied meaning to submit equally to everyone. Another possible interpretation is two sails or flags blowing in the wind. It represents the action/principle of Wind, that affects everyone.

***Yáng* 陽:** "sun, masculine principle, positive (electric)"

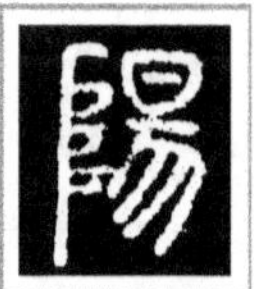

The image of a mound of earth or hill appears to the left of the image of the sun with its rays coming down, representing the sunny side of the hill. In the East Asian classics, *yáng* 陽 is coupled with *yīn* 陰 to give meaning to a system of interdependent couples or pairs such as light and dark, hot and cold, expanding and contracting, masculine and feminine.

***Yì (i)*易:** "easy, change"

This is an ancient image. *Yì* is the name of the *Classic of Change*, the *Yìjīng* 易精. The *Shuōwén jiězì* 《说文解字》 defines it as a kind of chameleon/ lizard (*yǎn tíng* 蝘蜓), while the oracle bone pictograms depict the changing light of the sun or moon.

***Yì (i)* 義:** "righteousness, justice,, right conduct"

The image above is the lamb or goat often used in sacrificial ceremonies, meaning "goodness." Below is the image of two swords clashing (or possibly a hand holding a sword.) The ideogram represents the justice that comes as a result of conflict resolution. *Yì* is one of the Confucian ideals.

***Yīn* 陰:** "overcast, cloudy, shady, negative (electric) feminine, moon, implicit, hidden, genitalia"

The image of a mound of earth or hill appears to the left of the image of a cloud, meaning the shady side of the hill. In the East Asian classics, *yīn* is coupled with *yáng* to give meaning to a system of interdependent couples such as light and dark, hot and cold, inside and outside, expanding and contracting, masculine and feminine.

Yōng **庸** "ordinary, common, everyday, usual"

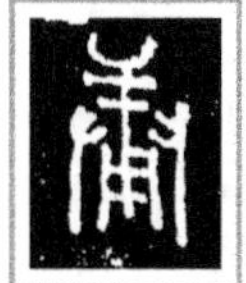

Thought to be the image of two hands on either side of a pestle *gēng* 庚 with a vessel *yōng* 用, between them symbolizing utility, usefulness, function. When combined with *Zhōng* 中: middle, central (see below), *Zhōngyōng* 中庸 refers to the Confucian "doctrine of the mean" or "middle way" (*zhōngyōng zhī dào* 中庸之道).

Yù **欲:** "desire, appetite, passion, long for, lust, greed"

On the right, is the image of a person exhaling, on left according to the *Shuōwén jiězì* 《说文解字》 (*Shouwen Dictionary*) is *gǔ* 谷, a valley. Perhaps this is a metaphor for the sighing sound of a valley stream, like a great exhale, or related to the heavy sigh one has when caught in wishful desire. Both Confucius and Lǎozǐ have much to say about the pitfalls and perils of excessive desire. See Appendix I: *Parting Words*.

Zhèn **振:** "to shake, rumble, shock, quake, excite, raise to action, one of the eight *bāguà* symbolizing thunder (☳)."

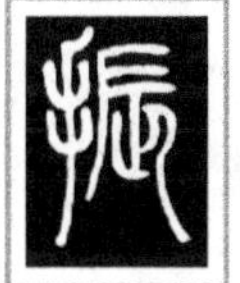

The image of a hand on the left next to a plow 辰 implied meaning: to disturb the ground like thunder. The action/principle of thunder – waking up life: two *yīn* lines above with a *yáng* rumbling below ☳.

***Zhōng* 中:** "center, centered, middle, in the midst of"

The image shows a vertical line bisecting a container or some say a kind of bullseye target. This character is also used for "China," indicating the so called "middle kingdom," or the central plain between the Yellow River (Huánghé 黃河) and the Yangtze (Cháng Jiāng長江).

***Zhéli* 哲理:** "Sage Principles"

***Zhé* 哲** "sage"

The image of a hand holding an axe, meaning to cut or carve, is placed above the mouth. This ideogram represents the sage or wise man who is said to be able to cut through confusion and entanglements with clarity and wisdom.

***Lǐ* 理:** "intrinsic order, inner principle, reason, logic, texture, science, grain of wood"

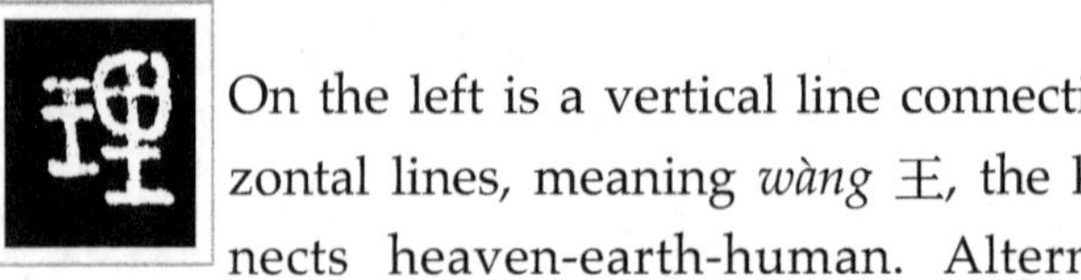

On the left is a vertical line connecting three horizontal lines, meaning *wàng* 王, the king who connects heaven-earth-human. Alternately this is thought to be jade. On the right is the field (*tián* 田**)** above the soil which by itself represents a unit of measure of an area, "the Chinese mile." According to Professor Cheng, *Lǐ* 理 is the organizing principle or constant that unifies the interactions of *yīn-yáng*, out of which comes *qì* 氣 and *xiàng* 象 (see Chapter 3).

Appendix III Notes:

---

317 Goblet words (*zhīyán* 卮言) see Wu (1982). *Chuang Tzu: World Philosopher at Play*, p. 34.

318 Descriptions of the seal characters (*zhuànshū* 篆書) are based on lively discussions Ed and I have had over many years, coupled with consultation from several resources: *Shuōwénjiězì* 《说文解字》 the Eastern Han dynasty etymological dictionary traditionally dated to 100 CE, as well as entries from HanziNet.org, Léon Wieger's *Chinese Characters: Their Origin, Etymology, History, Classification and Signification* (1965 edition), and works by Claude Larre, Elisabeth Rochat de la Vallée, and Sandra Schatzman (1968).

319 Callicott & Ames (1989). *Nature in Asian Traditions of Thought: Essays in Environmental Philosophy*, p. 119.

Appendix IV: Cheng Man-Ch'ing's Hand-Written *Sage Principles*

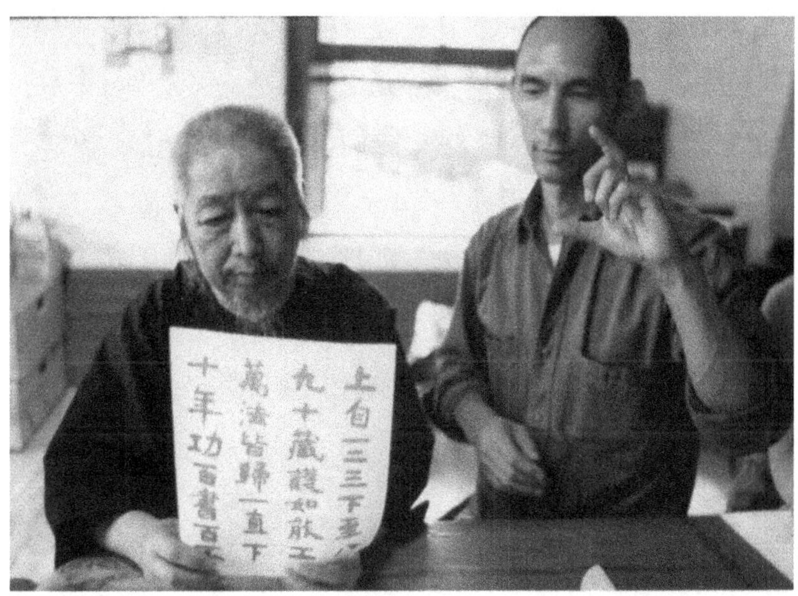

Cheng Man-Ch'ing Studying the Sage Masters & Ed Translating
Photo from Ed Young's Private Collection (possibly taken by Ken Van Sickle)

Preface by Cheng Man-ch'ing

翻譯節錄前哲要言之引言

中國之哲理貫乎三才含義至深近百餘年海
內外談及中國哲理者僅能涉及藩籬其故何
在以譯易與老子者多采王弼註弼註殊多謬
誤貽害匪淺茲節錄前哲要言如易與孔子之
繫辭以及黃帝內經與老子等書與吾太極拳運
動有息息相關者都一百七十五言然涉及人生哲
理而合乎生理及科學原理者殊多然中國之生
理學皆基於黃帝內經其理雖極透徹却甚
深奧學者如欲窮研此道非竭十分耐心純
取客觀態度不為功髯抱愚公移山之志非祗
乎暢達而不已茲將西方文字中所未有之字義先
加詳釋然後再將原文詳譯使讀者易乎明瞭
耳髯之希望能於學者萬人中得有一二人領略而
所願亦已足矣丙午冬日永嘉鄭曼髯識於紐約

Chapter 1: The Sage Principles

弗羅索非 Philosophy 中文譯作哲學應加修正說

中國稱黃帝曰聖哲書述唐虞稱濬哲文明孔子自稱哲人後人從未稱之為哲人學派希臘之蘇格拉底者所謂弗羅索非學派中文譯作哲學細閱其定義非常廣泛約言之為我愛智識追求真理及其流派之演變除於生理及宗教外甚至謂世界一切事之与物及宇宙萬有之原理原則之學也以此說法加以澈底考驗其理由予以批評与分析直是文學趨乎科學化之途徑如以中文翻譯祇可作智人學派或簡稱為智學可耳若視同中國之哲理則圓鑿方枘不相入矣茲將以上三點之哲理約畧言之一黃帝稱聖哲又將老聃合而稱之曰黃老哲理以無為為宗二唐堯虞舜之濬哲文明易繫辭曰黃帝堯舜垂衣裳而天下治此猶以堯舜繼起黃帝之無為也三孔子自稱哲人弟子讚稱謂天縱之將聖

又稱之曰夫子其聖然乎孔子曰聖則吾不能繞此以上相較聖与哲之荅案可比諸道之与德也道始制有名猶如聖也德資生之實猶如哲也孔子之不居聖人之名誠已具有哲人之實以此可知聖与哲之不同正猶名之与實耳然而孔子本立人之道曰仁与義以克己為體中庸為用而達其修齊治平之道親九族而昭明百姓之教此即孔子哲人之學也老聃則不然曰吾愚人之心也哉以絕學棄智為用此乃中國之哲理俱甚簡明不同歐西弗羅索非學派之繁複也且孔子有言曰何多哉君子不多也倘必要講通中西文化應自正名為始故說明中國之哲理如此不可視同弗羅索非之說也

Chapter 2: 175 Words of the Sages

易曰君子終日乾々夕惕若厲无咎

易書名曰述也始創於伏羲氏成於周代所述者曰理曰氣曰象三者含有交易不易變易之義君子謂才德超人之學者

又曰天行健君子以自強不息

又引證說天之行動至健且無休息故君子效法焉

孔子則曰易有太極而生兩儀兩儀生四象四象生八卦

孔子名丘字仲尼乃從古學人中之出類拔萃者是以稱為至聖先師

謂易有太極太極乃包舉理氣象三者之原則而未分布之象徵

又曰剛柔相摩八卦相盪

剛柔者陰與陽也八卦易有附圖相摩者互相迫切著摩抄也相盪者乃運化而推移也

又曰剛柔相推而變化

剛與柔相接觸而推移則變化生焉以所謂交易變易之理可以見焉甚至不易之理亦已寓於其中焉

岐伯則曰夫道者祛老而全形精神內守病安從來是以志閑而少欲

岐伯者乃黃帝師也在公元前二十有七世紀授黃帝以醫學而成答問曰素問內經

夫道即所謂卻老全形之修養法則也精神內守使不外馳而消失是以病無從由虛隙可襲也

又曰筋脉和同骨髓堅固氣血皆從

筋脉和同不見露骨髓堅固已至填精補髓之候則氣血皆已相從矣兩者乃為返老還童之實證

附注

筋脈和同筋以行氣屬於陽脈以行血屬於陰筋猶電線脈猶水管得能和同者正謂氣血相調陰陽相濟

黃帝則曰陽氣者精則養神柔則養筋聖人傳精神服天氣而通神明

黃帝軒轅氏古帝名滅蚩尤而有天下為吾中華民族之始祖

陽氣者生生不已之氣也精者華五臟分泌之精華且精足方可以養神是即精氣為神之說也

柔柔和也筋喜柔和而得養筋如剛強乾燥便如草木枯槁則肝臟必至硬化可知矣因筋者即屬於肝系故也

老子則曰虛其心實其腹弱其志強其骨

老子姓老名聃謂姓李者誤也予另著有老聃傳可供參考為周藏室史著有道德經五千言

虛其心者是置心於無為境界之內乃氣與丹田相守丹田即藏精之室另有分釋見釋精條

實其腹即氣丹田志乃氣之帥也志之所至氣隨至之因志向好強必使之柔弱始能降於丹田然後方可以得強其骨也

又曰天下之至柔馳騁天下之至堅

天下之至柔者未有能超過風與水也如能收斂其氣力鍥而不舍則古有謂風過銅摩水滴石穿及其積力之大甚至排山倒海世界又有何物得能禦之也

又曰專氣致柔能嬰兒乎

如能專氣積於丹田通於膜達於筋脈可使和同而致柔一若嬰兒焉

Chapter 3: Lǐ, Qì, Xiàng 理氣象 and the Eight Trigram Bāguà 八卦 Sequence

一即理理即一也、一之周流為無極、附圖
是為無極、無極者包舉大氣而已、是為混沌
附圖 是為混沌乃清濁未分之時、清濁始
分是為太極、附圖 此乃太極未判之時、太極
既判則清濁分、是為一生二、附圖 之
為太極生兩儀、○為氣未為天◎為象[illegible]為地
是理乃以一理貫通天地之氣象也理者乃
天地原始之道理也先天地而已具傳天
地或有時而毀滅惟此道理則終不滅也

Chapter 4: Hún and Pò 魂魄

魂与魄

老子有謂營魄抱一能無離乎營在內經為營衛營則屬於血衛則屬於氣所謂營魄者既魂魄也因魂為血之氣魄為氣之氣猶熱氣也血常降及其死則反之而上升為魂氣常升及死其則反之為下降而為魄魂魄不能抱一是謂離也曾子曰陽之精氣曰神即氣之熱氣也陰之精氣曰靈即謂血之氣也魂与魄之別為此而已矣可見魂魄離則神靈与軀殼脫離而謂之死魂与魄聚則為鬼獨離其軀殼不能用也魂与魄之說不知西方國家如何說法然鬼之所謂人所不易見者或在半信半疑之中耳此說無他用意惟謂氣与血皆屬於物質物質永為不滅者不过中國不但只說不滅且有其定名以供西方之哲学家其細審察之也魂魄之離也其作用有限若謂魂魄抱一其用可勝言哉亦希近代医學家注意之焉

Chapter 5: Essence-Spirit and Blood-Breath
Jīngshén Xuèqì 精神血氣

釋精

精內經謂萃五臟六腑之精華歸乎腎而謂之曰精西醫謂一滴精乃四十滴血之所構成者男女媾精之時必經氣海氣海即丹田每關元而後瀉出故罵人謂男女之事無節制者精從下流而不禁謂之下流聖哲如黃帝老子之流不獨具有節制而已且欲有以補益之也是謂曰鍊精鍊精化炁乃是東方哲學上之第一步功夫從而釋之如下

精足便可使神旺此常人皆可得而能也瀉之過多者不在此例黃老為修養家之始創者所謂鍊精化炁之法其主要之處即是氣海一名丹田又名藏精之室丹田者即煉丹之田其位置在腹內臍下一寸三分與臍近去脊較遠約十之三與七相比以心與氣相守丹田乃是以血氣之氣凝注丹田心即以心靈之心亦與之相守不離丹田然後以呼吸引空氣亦灌注丹田使丹田所必經之精留注以心與氣相守之鍥而不舍久之可使精暖而亦化炁此氣之熱力猶電力然由尾閭骨節間越過輭筋透達骨內因骨無其他隙縫傳入之熱氣猶烟霧籠罩骨中俟熱退時則凝為流質如汗水待冷則流質又化為固體如極薄之玻璃紙一層貼於骨中是為骨髓積久則盈上達於腦腦為髓海髓滙於海則鍊精化炁之法如此而已

Chapter 6: The System of Tendons, Channels, and Membrane Networks 筋脈与膜膈之系统

筋脈与膜膈之系統

中國医學將行氣之系統注重於此四部门曰筋曰脈曰膜曰膈其主要之原理正為西医所未曾注意者即乎在一氣字而已。其所謂氣乃率血而行倘不言氣則血液之循環失其主動之作用矣。是以太極拳極端求鬆之與柔者即注重乎運氣之作用耳。故氣沈丹田行乎膜而通乎膈達乎筋而溢脈不独使血液之循環已耳五臟六腑及各器官皆於氣血向從之冲和狀態中得舒適之運動。若以西医方面而言不拉斯不拉斯脫中间之空位称為盧门不拉斯發育而成胎其中空位減少以漸消失者此盧门即所謂氣海亦称為丹田即西医所謂葛雷特屋門也又為全体膜膈之中心耳人之中心全体及乎皮膚未有不関乎膜膈灌輸之作用其源即在乎丹田耳。

Chapter 7: Yīn-Yáng, Five Phases and the Five Organs 陰陽五行五臟

陰陽与五行之分釋

陰陽与五行乃中西哲理之与科学相隔閡惟之焦点与中国哲理与科学能相貫通者即賴陰陽与五行為橋樑耳而西方之哲学与科学有所隔閡者惜未能了解此橋樑之作用故特詳為分釋之陰陽乃天地男女雌雄牝牡寒熱燥濕以及萬物之有兩种不同性能之類悉以陰陽二字包括而總代表之亦猶数学之有代数而代為医学家之術語在中国哲学与科学上乃最重之關鍵譬猶近代之電学家及原子学家如核子之分析至窮極不得再分時猶具有兩种不同性能存在除名之曰陰陽二字之外尚猶有他之切當者如無線電亦有陰陽兩种性能之相求相应亦可以通達者故陰之為●陽之為○乃五千年前伏羲氏之創始作易畫八卦時根據上古之河圖洛書而明其致理故孔子易繫辭有謂河出圖洛出書聖人則之即指此耳五行者乃金木水火土為天地所產生五种特殊物質且具有相生相尅之性能亦洛書天一生水地二生火之原則以相推其至理而致成易經故取五行以相佐陰陽不独猶数字有代数而已且兼代萬物之性能与相生尅之作用盡致毫厘不爽是其倖言此物比方物質当然是科学若以其用言以物質之性能与生尅原則取以比喻哲理而使哲理不致空虛其实俱不離有氣与象耳此之謂哲理而誠未離乎科学也是之謂昔日之哲理即證今日之科学今日科学之進境亦即昔日之哲理也然以此之分釋亦不过僅其原則若必欲解其妙用之实者非潛心窮究不易得也

Chapter 8: The Heart and Spine

釋　心

心在說文六書乃象形之字是即為形之君亦曰神明之主也

心為五臟之一五臟乃心肝脾肺腎也內經謂心之性能屬火火即五行之一五行乃金木水火土之五種性能取以直接代表五臟之相生相尅之生理與作用以其有事實證明容易了解此亦猶數學之代數已目可見中國之醫學在五千年前已已具有最高深之科學原理未可忽視也以下先分釋五行之生尅五行之金乃斧鋸之類可以伐木即金尅木木之根向地下伸展即木尅土土可吸收水份即土尅水水可以滅火即水尅火火可以鎔化五金即火尅金此自然相尅之理從之釋相生　金得溫度便生潮濕經煅煉必先出水鎔液亦猶水然即金生水水不論江海皆能生草木且木又非得水不得即水生木木至千年不火自焚牟嶋子紅木林中頗多腹部自成焦炭可以見矣又鑽木可以取火即木生火火所焚餘之物均為灰土即火生土土中所產生者具有五金即土生金此亦自然相生之理然在人之五臟生尅之原理與五行生尅之原理悉無分別可說絲絲入扣此即易之天地人一理之憑據悉不出乎陰陽五行而已在天即為日月五星在地即為動植五行在人即為男女五倫（五倫即君臣父子夫婦兄弟朋友也）然皆不出乎陰陽五行之理耳惟五臟生尅之理與五行相並論其詳已見乎內經非一二言可了茲所釋者惟心臟其餘概從簡略其詳請參考內經

心臟之性能

按照美國衛生局報告、國內患心臟病致死者、平均每兩分鐘喪失一人、其嚴重性可想而知、茲擬將中國醫學家、對於心臟病之分析、及生理之說明、殊有異同、茲略舉一二以供病患者及醫師之參考、未知有裨補於萬一否、并希並世之醫學家、有以正之、則人類之幸也、

中國醫學、對於心臟之治理、即以五臟配合五行、以相生相尅循環之原理、為主旨、視直接之治理、猶若次之、故其用藥、以君臣佐使相配合、而以一藥獨用為誡、可見其對五臟之統籌、尚平治之方也、夫心配五行屬火、其詳已見上說、肝木生心火、猶母也、脾土猶子也、腎水猶仇敵也、肺金直受其尅制耳、必先審其損益之因、然後究其有餘或不足之實、則斷其安危之機、決其截補之法、此之謂全體大治也、萬一診察其命根已絕、則不立方投藥、必告以另請高明、故華陀所謂、祇能治病、不能救命、此中醫之治療、乃盡人事已耳、惟急欲究其損益之鉅者腎與肝也、餘臟暫可緩論、然而人莫不飲食也、飲食不能離乎五味、故以五味、參與五臟與五行、取

其切近、得以申述・期其易諭也、心之本味為苦、茶味苦、酒味亦尚苦、咖啡與香烟皆苦味也、人多酷好之、而不肯舍、尤其如鴉片與嗎啡、乃至苦、且極毒、人皆知其為身體之禍害、且有舍命而好之者、是以心之有所嗜也、且至於是、以其与生理相近耳、不獨心之於味、其切要有如此、餘臟亦皆然也、惟所尚之味不同耳、脾喜甜、肺喜辣、腎喜鹹、肝喜酸、此亦各臟之本味也、倘有人喜食鹹味過多者、其腎臟必獨旺盛、是則腎水獨旺、有滅心火之虞、乃心臟受其損害也、抑有人喜食酸味過多者、其肝臟必獨旺盛、是則肝木獨旺、有生心火之益、乃心臟受其利也、此之謂相生相尅之損益、其積習非一朝一夕之故、有數十年、或終身者、其致病之因、由來已久、久則不易平治也、然人苟欲強其心者、必須於日常生活中多加注意、則易於獲益也、譬如肝乃益心猶母也、應如何始能善護肝木、余以為除飲食之酸辣二味善為運用外、第一要求寬和舒展、抑鬱局促非所宜也、因筋絡百脈、悉屬於肝、正要如木之枝幹條達扶疎、尤忌憤怒、倘能加以輕鬆柔婉之運動、如莊周所謂熊經鳥伸、作舒筋活絡、自強不息、使氣血自然調暢、則尤為佳妙、此外直接求心臟之安寧與修養、則不出乎率性任真四字而已、因心之性能為火、火乃光明磊落之象、亦猶赤日當空之概、稍有雲霧蔽之則晦、故書有云、作偽則心勞日拙、此言最明心理之樞要、人之作偽、未有不昧其真、而害性能、正猶雲霧之蔽日、而喪其心理、惡得安寧、又何修養之可言也、進之欲求安心之法、無如潛心下氣、寧靜澹泊、已耳、倘致心臟失其平衡、或直接有他種病患發生、必須審其原因由、然後加以補救、亦已盡其人事、如其性能已至枯竭、亦可以休矣、若必求掉換一他人之心臟、希圖苟活、縱有通神之技、可能改造其心臟、則其餘四臟亦早已報廢、雖可苟延殘喘、終歸烏有、而可惜其妙技矣、余甚以顏回早夭孔明不壽、未能盡其妙用、殊為可惜、倘能易其心臟、得以苟活、我必謂已非顏回與孔明矣、又何足貴、又何足惜、人所貴有其靈氣、用完則已矣、生死末事耳、猶稻之早熟早收、晚熟晚穫、既有收穫、餘亦猶草之根莖、棄之可矣、所以欲求良醫之良治者、不過欲遂其天年亦已足矣、未知有識者、以我言為何如

心膂並重

內經以任督同舉書亦嘗以心膂並稱而尤以道家對於心膂與修養之關係言之詳矣太極拳乃內家拳也宋末張真人三丰祖述黃老無為然後有為之說合周易理氣象之義以演成究其要者仍不出乎任督任督居奇經八脈之首任心主之督膂主之膂即屬於脊以體分而言之則膂為體心為用合而言之則心膂交而體用全矣太極拳之所以超乎其他拳術及運動者亦以是之所致也心為人一身之主聖賢之學之要曰求其放心禪者曰主人翁在家否主人翁者心也猶道家所謂心膂交者大同小異耳然同工亦能各有其所長惟太極拳卻有進乎是焉正有所謂不如見諸行事之為深切著明矣吾以是而有心膂並重之論作欲以明乎有體斯有用之實者矣心者非謂肉團之心也乃心靈之心也心靈之心與肉團之心本非二亦非一也即肉團之心之能有作用而靈一切者乃心靈之心也膂脊骨也脊二十四節為人體最多節之主骨五臟六腑繫焉五體軀幹賴以支撐此猶餘事耳談修養與衛生之道舍此皆末事也太極拳主務本之功亦在於斯而已初學入門者即以心與氣相守於丹田勿忘勿助此即所謂求其放心及主人翁之在家也久之氣自能歷乎尾閭沖開夾脊度乎玉枕而達乎顛頂降於丹田此即任督通而心膂交矣然此非一朝一夕之故尤不可牽強純其自然苟能臻此則不獨太極拳之有登峯造極之望其精神庶乎所以不死矣長生祛病更無論矣雖然心膂難言之矣有學識及修養者固不乏人如前哲所謂心傳及正心與不動心之說誠者日月經天自能取法何待贅述惟膂之一字意猶未盡約而言之古人所謂正襟危坐者此修養之事也危字之解不一皆未敢直作危險之危字解予謂危坐者確有危險之實存乎其間脊多節若串珠然累疊而起稍不經意則傾側或曲西而倒矣則不復有力得能支撐其軀幹矣知其所以然弗使漸為不振由萎靡而致為病也故有臨深履薄之戒曰正襟危坐正則不病矣危則恐其易乎不正以致其病也余乃為留意太極拳者告曰豎起脊樑豎起者正若串珠累疊串令其傾側而已若緊張矜持矯枉過正皆病也只要知其為危可矣無以加矣

Chapter 9: The Dāntián 丹田

丹田

四十多年前当我寫太極拳十三篇時友人專松兄告知有法蘭西師從人体解剖垂二十年才發現道家所謂丹田之所在在腹部腸与腸相連之網膜中有一若囊者惟運動及武術家則囊之度独厚甚至大可容拳当時以其最新發現未證明我國所謂丹田之説有根據也丹田在黄帝内経称為氣海老子黄庭經称為丹田均説得非常清楚西医又称為奧門屯且謂此囊能上下抵禦外来之襲擊者舉例謂当腹部解剖時此網膜能遮蓋刀割之處又盲腸發炎此囊也能盡量遮蓋發炎之處謂其有伸縮能力下圖為標準西医究寧漢生理教科書中解釋惟西医僅知其形態与部位及動力已耳而不知有氣作用故特別徹底作詳細之解釋耳

丹田与黄庭

按西医之生理學在人体之臟腑内有二部份謂不起作用一在腹部腸之膜網中有一若囊者名之曰葛蕾特屋門屯一在腰後近脊即傍脾与胰子之間有一空隙係黄色者亦謂不起作用又名之曰勅賽屋門屯在我國医学及道家指此二者謂在人体上起最重要之作用一葛蕾特屋門屯即名之曰丹田一勅賽屋門屯即名之黄庭雖名称不同部位則一也然其形体及顏色俱無以異而决無疑義者乃有至理存焉茲約略分釋其作用中医注重氣化之作用西医尚未注意及此中医在黄帝時已作内経垂五千年老子從黄帝而言道乃著有黄庭經俱極言丹田与黄庭之妙用有涉及陰陽与五行之至理且中国生理學之根據不能離乎是也此有關人生性命之本非窮不易了解茲不过考證中西医学名称之異同与作用之有懸殊已耳

Chapter 10: The Physiology of a Baby
嬰兒之生理

嬰兒之生理

岐伯曰筋脈和同骨髓堅固氣血皆從老子曰專氣致柔能嬰兒乎今得此圖形卻可作哲理與生理相對之實證其奧妙正待詳細之分析也一從此X光透視嬰兒之骨骼與成人之骨骼大異在每骨節處處見其肢體骨節之距離皆相去甚大全憑筋絡之維繫得以貫串而動作可見筋絡和同之作用極大一其氣血充足其整体有如皮球任其跌扑不致損傷可見其骨髓之堅固也所謂專氣致柔雖年老之人也可以有還童之望者正賴其乎養氣之功得能玩此妙理可無疑義也

Chapter 11: The Adult Skeleton 成人骨骼

成人骨骼

由此圖可見骨節之每節均已啣接
緊湊与嬰兒之骨節正相反即是筋脈
乾燥不得和同骨髓漸見消耗不
得堅固將成枯槁矣此亦已成剛強
壯強狀態不是柔弱之嬰兒可比故老
子曰柔弱者生之徒也剛強者死之徒也

Chapter 12: Explanation of the Sacrum 尾閭骨之解釋

141

尾閭骨之解釋

尾閭為脊錐骨之末節即另有五小節組成者以上有八個孔為兩相聚是以名之曰閭閭者里中之門形容其
聚也惟此八孔之作用極為重要在人身生理上成一樞機故名之曰尾閭不可輕視此尾閭之八孔可以引
之精氣入於脊骨中此為第一關漸轉變為骨髓越過玉枕骨為第二關達乎顛頂為泥丸乃第三關此三關
髓之作用俱已詳見以上精與氣之二條中恕不贅即中西醫所謂所謂血液循環及內分泌之作用皆不及
氣為髓之重要據西醫克寧漢醫學教科書於九十二頁開始便說尾閭於古時已認為身體恢復之種子及其
典內之解釋恢復乃由一不增之地部升到一個強壯之狀況由此可知尾閭之重要中西醫學有可互為證
即如此類可惜此種生理之深奧意義近乎哲理未易了解好像在近代醫學中已被遺棄或者視同神秘恐
生理上受莫大之損失並希望未來之医學有以注意及之

成人骨骼

由此圖可見骨節之每節均已啣接緊湊與嬰兒之骨節正相反即是節脹乾燥不得和同骨髓漸見消耗不
將成枯槁矣此亦已成剛強狀態不是柔弱之嬰兒可比故老子有曰柔弱者生之徒也剛強者死之徒也

CHAPTER XII

尾閭骨之解釋

尾閭為脊錐骨之末節，另有五小節即組成者，
以上有八箇孔，為兩行相聚，是以名之曰閭，閭
者里中之門也，形容其多户相聚也，惟此八孔之作
用，極為重要，在人身陰上，成一樞機，故名之曰
尾閭，不可輕視，此為第一關，此尾閭之八孔，可以藉引導精
氣入於脊骨中，轉變為骨髓，而精
此節已詳言之
越過玉枕骨為第二關，達乎顛
頂為泥丸宮，乃第三關，此三關皆精髓之作用，此已詳見
以上精與氣之二條件，絕不贅，即中西醫
之所謂血液之循環，及內分泌之作用，皆不及
此精化氣為髓之重要，故西醫未寧、漢醫

學教科書於九十三頁開始、便說尾閭於古時已認為身體恢復之種子，及韋氏大字典內之解釋、恢復、乃由一不增之地部，升到一個強壯之狀況，由此可知尾閭之重要，中西醫學有可互為證明者之處、即為此類、可惜此種生理之深奧意義、近乎哲理、未易了解、好像在近代醫學中、已被遺棄、或者視同神秘、因恐在人類之生理上、發生莫大之損失、並希望未來之醫學有以注意及之、

Chapter 13: The Mystery of Hormones

荷爾蒙之究竟

世界醫學上屢見荷爾蒙神妙之學說據所謂帶刺激性之內分泌有特別之效用及能傳達總神經節之本體與核又稱為內分泌腺與胰臟中之細胞所產生此化學物對生物機構中有妙極之效用等語均未有確定之分解但僅知其神妙卻未知其所以為神妙茲將其與中國醫學有脗合之處者特標而出之至於鄙人有未敢苟同之論亦姑從而舉之以供參考對於根據及出處另詳附注根據全体十五腺之所產生荷爾蒙與中國醫學之任督二脈相通及道家之河車倒運正相脗合其次第與始末附見圖註.其作用悉照照中國定義為之分釋以供世界醫學家之參考任督二脈相通與河車倒運已見前鍊化氣篇茲亦附圖註餘不復贅其次第當以腎上腺為主体即標以1.腎上腺乃本上古之洛書天一生水之說質五行屬水乃已越過河車之第一關之尾閭亦已見上說 2.為腦下垂体乃河車之第二關玉枕 3.松果腺將近河車第三關泥丸之甲狀腺及甲狀旁腺則已越過河車之第三關泥丸已下含津玉液矣金津玉液二脈絡在舌根下 4.胸腺為十二重樓已屬任脈 5.為胰腺屬於脾 6.為睾丸也卵巢為任脈之終矣此約為十五點其次第絲毫不爽其程序與始末亦不能越乎此是為內泌有源之主流惟其名稱與中醫不同其實即津液也津液乃陰陽之分不止一种之分泌各臟腑不同也津屬於陽分潤於氣之所產生者液屬於陰潤乎血之所產生者細辨之各有作用與來源及其程序與始末而知其本能得予以名稱惟津稀薄液較濃厚津行氣管可以由肺直入膜腸液則行食管入脾胃分五臟是以總名之曰津液乃有陰陽之分所謂荷爾蒙之有刺激性之內分泌即與內分泌有所異同又據謂荷爾蒙之細胞有可能直入血球者或有半數不可能入血球者以此可證荷爾蒙之有陰陽陰屬於血陽屬氣惟氣乃率血而行當然可以入血球或有半數可入血球者其半屬於氣不可以入血球者乃屬乎血血球與血球類也以無化生作用故不相入也在中醫之金津玉液於人身体中為惟一由化生之主要活力除所謂荷爾蒙具有奇妙作用外無可比擬者故予以上二點反覆申述其產生之原動力與位置之次第及血球與細胞之分合以及一切之作用而非息息相關可見了無疑義矣至於近代發明荷爾蒙之分劑由分析人体本有之荷爾蒙與動植物生物体上之荷爾蒙相對比而擷取其作用原不背乎

科學此亦了無疑義惟他種物体上之荷爾蒙增益人体上作用必有乖戾於自然
之生理致有所損益則不得不徹底加以窮究茲舉數事望商榷焉 1.人体之荷爾蒙
原有自能化生之力量倘稍有虧損者何不使其自力更生之力量以資挽救若確無自生
能力然後暫施代替品以冀續絕未為晚也今不此之思直認攫取他種荷爾蒙以
為靈藥竊非良医之良治也 2.倘人体之荷爾蒙已致虧損不过其活力暫形衰退已耳不
致驟患大病茲取他種荷爾蒙填補往往致大病或速其死亡其故何在寧容緩究
乎吾觀動植物所需要之活力不一定是人所需要之活力人之虧損荷爾蒙不一定取動植物
之荷爾蒙可以填補以其種類與性質及陰陽之作用不同未能完全相合然不獨此一意
而已以人体之產生之荷爾蒙原為有所需要今以有过多代替品則人体中當然不須再事產生
然虧損是病過多亦是病况以不得其法之填補欲以使十五腺上下堵截不通新陳
代謝則失其循環之作用矣此外如男人誤服女用之荷爾蒙漸致變性如乳房隆起或生
殖器萎縮之類女人如誤用男用荷爾蒙其變性亦猶是如乳房癟塌髭鬚猛茁之類象
徵頓見以此可證荷爾蒙本有陰陽之別亦可證其效用之神是以知荷爾蒙即金津玉
液無疑金津玉液之分布津可直達六腑液可直入五臟皆可增益臟腑之精華亦猶
十五腺荷爾蒙之增益活力也然臟腑之精華充滿有餘力則均滙歸於腎以構成
男女之陽精與陰精之原料已耳所謂荷爾蒙之作用妙極者即如此而已是為荷爾蒙
之事实如此未為过也况人体上除此並無第二种活力能具此作用也科学医学一也如
離乎实情实事又豈足称為医学科学哉中國之医学涉及哲理以其学理过于透澈且
無一不符乎自然自然之理实難言其玄妙予不过憑五千年來前哲遺言得以分釋其所脗
合之點已耳茲據生命科学一書所称生活科学與新陳代謝剛才開始從荷爾蒙之研
究此誠不失為学者之懸鵠不禁感歎茲亦不辭繁冗必欲將此意作精審切實
之解釋冀使世界好学者讀之或亦易乎了解吾前哲之医理可作進一步之究竟不致為
深奧学理有所隔閡庶中西医学得有溝通之望達全人類保健之至幸想高明者
聞之或不以吾言為河漢

己酉立夏後三日 鄭曼髯初稿

荷爾蒙之究竟

世界医學上屢見荷爾蒙神妙之學說據所謂帶刺激性之內分泌有特別之效用及能傳達總神經節之本體與核又稱為內分泌腺與其腸中之細胞所產生此化學物對生物機構中有妙極之效用等語向未有確定之分解但僅知其神妙卻未知其所以為神妙茲將其與中國醫學有脗合之處者特標而出之至於鄙人有未敢苟同之論亦姑從而舉之以供參考又指今根據及出處另詳附注根據全体十五腺之所產生荷爾蒙與中國醫學之任督二脈相通及道家之河車倒運正相脗合其次第與始末附見圖註其作用悉照中國医定數為之分釋以供世界医學家之參考任督二脈相通與河車倒運已見前錄化氣篇茲亦附圖註餘不復贅其次第當以腎上腺為主体即標以1.腎上腺乃合上古之洛書天一生水之說腎五行屬水乃已越過河車之第一関之尾閭亦已見上說之為腦下垂体乃河車之第二関玉枕3.松果腺將近河車第三関泥丸至甲狀腺及甲狀旁腺則已越過河車之第三関泥丸已下金津玉液矣金津玉液二脈絡在舌根下4.胸腺為十二重樓已屬任脈5.為胰腺屬於脾6.為男睪丸女卵巢為任脈之終点此約為十五点其次第絲毫不爽其程序與始末亦不能越乎此是為內分泌有源之主流惟其名稱與中医不同其實即津液也津液乃陰陽之分不止一種之分泌各臟腑不同也津屬於陽分関於氣之所產生者液屬於陰分関乎血之所產生者細辨之各有其作用與來源及其程序與始末而知其今能得予以名稱惟津稀薄液較濃厚津行氣管可以由肺直入膜膈液則行食管入脾胃分布五臟是以總名之曰津液乃有陰陽之分所謂荷爾蒙之有刺激性之內分泌即於內分泌有所異同又據謂荷爾蒙之細胞有可能直入血球者或有半數不可能入血球者以此可證荷爾蒙之有陰陽陰屬於血陽屬氣惟氣乃率血而行当然可以入血球或有半數可入血球者其半屬於氣不可以入血球者乃屬乎血血球與血球類也以無化生作用故不相入也在中医之金津玉液於人身体中為惟一由化生之主要活力除所謂荷爾蒙具有奇妙作用外無可比擬者故予以上二点反覆申述其產生之原動力與位置之次第及血球與細胞之分合以及一切之作用而非息息相関可見了無疑義矣至於近代發明荷爾蒙之方劑由分析人体本有之荷爾蒙與動植物之物体上之荷爾蒙相对比而擷取其作用原不背乎

References

Ahmad, S., Isbatan, A., Chen, S., Dudek, S. M., Minshall, R. D., and Chen, J. (2024). *The Interplay of Heart Failure and Lung Disease: Clinical Correlations, Mechanisms, and Therapeutic Implications. Journal of Respiratory Biology and Translational Medicine, 1*(4).

Alhababi, N., Magnus, M. C., Drake, M. J., Fraser, A., and Joinson, C. (2021). *The Association Between Constipation and Lower Urinary Tract Symptoms in Parous Middle-aged Women: A Prospective Cohort Study. Journal of Women's Health, 30*(8), 1171–1181. doi:10.1089/jwh.2020.8727

Ames, R. T., and Hall, D. L. (2001). *Focusing the Familiar: a Translation and Philosophical Interpretation of the Zhongyong*. Honolulu, HI: University of Hawai'i Press.

_____., and _____.. (2003). *Dao De Jing "Making This Life Significant": A Philosophical Translation*. New York, NY: Ballantine Books.

Ames, R. T. (2015). *The Great Commentary (Dàzhuàn 大傳) and Chinese Natural Cosmology. International Communication of Chinese Culture, 2*(1), 1–18. https://doi.org/10.1007/s40636-015-0013-2

Andrews, J. F., and Shen, K. (2016). *The Modernization of Chinese Art: The Shanghai Art College, 1913–1937*. Leuven, Belgium: Leuven University Press.

Benias, P. C., and Thiess, D. (2018). *The New Tissue That Could Change Medicine. Scientific American, 318*(5), 64–69.

Benias, P. C., Wells, R. G., Sackey-Aboagye, B., Klavan, H., Reidy, J., Buonocore, D., and Fuchs, B. C. (2018). *Structure and Distribution of an Unrecognized Interstitium in Human Tissues. Scientific Reports, 8*, 4947. doi:10.1038/s41598-018-23062-6

Berthon, B. S., and Wood, L. G. (2015). *Nutrition and Respiratory Health—Feature Review. Nutrients, 7*(3), 1618–1643. doi:10.3390/nu7031618

Buyadaa, O., Wolfe, R., Tonkin, A. M., et al. (2025). *Kidney Function and Risk of Heart Failure in Older Adults: Findings from a Prospective Cohort Study. Heart*. Advance online publication. https://doi.org/10.1136/heart-2025-XXXXXX

Callicott, J. B., and Ames, R. T. (1989). *Nature in Asian Traditions of Thought: Essays in Environmental Philosophy*. Albany, NY: State University of New York Press.

Capdevila, J. A., Martínez-Vázquez, J. M., Almirante, B., and Hernandez, A. (1990). *Liver Alterations in Acute Pneumonia. Archives of Internal Medicine, 150*(10), 2206–2209.

Chan, P. (2017). *The Making of a Modern Art World: Institutionalisation and Legitimisation of Guohua in Republican Shanghai.* Boston, MA: Brill.

Chen, X., Cui, J., Li, R., Norton, R., Park, J., Kong, J., and Yeung, A. (2019). *Dao Yin (a.k.a. Qigong): Origin, Development, Potential Mechanisms, and Clinical Applications. Evidence-Based Complementary and Alternative Medicine, 2019,* Article ID 3705120. doi:10.1155/2019/3705120

Cheng, M.C. (1950). *Zhengzi taiji quan shisan pian* [Thirteen treatises].

_____., Lo, B. P. J., and Inn, M (1985). *Cheng Tzu's Thirteen Chapters on T'ai-chi Ch'uan*. Berkeley, CA: Blue Snake Books.

_____., and Gibbs, T. (1981). *Lao Tzu: My Words Are Very Easy to Understand: Lectures on the Tao Teh Ching*. Berkley, CA: North Atlantic Books.

Cryan, J. F., O'Riordan, K. J., Cowan, C. S. M., Sandhu, S. M. E., Bastiaanssen, T. F. R., Boehme, M., and Dinan, T. G. (2018). *The Neuroendocrinology of the Microbiota–gut–brain axis: A Behavioural Perspective. Frontiers in Neuroendocrinology, 51,* 80–101. doi:10.1016/j.yfrne.2018.04.002

Cui, J., Qian, C., and Liu, Y. (2025). *Effect of Tai Chi on Bone Mineral Density in Middle-aged and Older Adults: A Meta-Analysis. Orthopedic Reviews, 17,* 125422. https://doi.org/10.52965/001c.125422

Davis, B. (2004). *The Taiji Quan Classics: An Annotated Translation*. Berkeley, CA: Blue Snake Books.

Ellis, A., and Wiseman, N. (1989). *Grasping the Wind: An Exploration into the Meaning of Chinese Acupuncture Point Names*. Brookline, MA: Paradigm Publications.

Fu, S., Lin, F., and Vankeerberghen, G. (2025). *The Great Commentary on the Documents Classic / Shangshu dazhuan* 大傳. Seattle, WA: University of Washington Press.

Fox, W. (1984). *Deep Ecology: A New Philosophy of Our Time?* The Ecologist, *14,* 194–200.

Gibbs, T. (1985, June). *Cheng Tzu: Master of the Five Excellences.* Full Circle, 1(2), 13–21.

Guo, Y., Zhao, J., and Zhang, Q. (2018). *Beneficial effects of Qigong Wuqinxi in the iImprovement of Chronic Low Back Pain, Physical Fitness, and Quality of Life in the Elderly*. Evidence-Based Complementary and Alternative Medicine, 2018, Article ID 3235950. doi:10.1155/2018/3235950

Hadi, H., Di Vincenzo, A., Vettor, R., & Rossato, M. (2020). *Relationship Between Heart Disease and Liver Disease: A Two-way Street.* Cells, 9(3), 567. doi:10.3390/cells9030567

Hiss, A. (1973, October 29). *"Hold It!"* The New Yorker, 35–36.

Hoizey, D. (1993). *A History of Chinese Medicine.* Edinburgh, UK: Edinburgh University Press.

Huang, A. (1998). *The Complete I Ching: The Definitive Translation by the Taoist Master Alfred Huang.* Rochester, VT: Inner Traditions International.

Kircher, K. F. (1987). How the sacrum got its name. *JAMA, 258*(3), 325. https://doi.org/10.1001/jama.1987.03400030041020

Larre, C., and Rochat de la Vallée, E. (1991). *The Heart.* Monkey Press.

_____. (2003). *The Extraordinary Fu.* Brookline, MA: Monkey Press.

Legge, J. (1879). *The Sacred Books of the East, vol. III.* London, UK: Oxford University Press/Clarendon Press.

_____. (1882). *The Sacred Books of the East vol. XVI.* London, UK: Oxford University Press/Clarendon Press.

_____. (1883). *The Chinese Classics.* New York, NY: John B Alden.

Lowenthal, W. (1991). *There Are No Secrets: Professor Cheng Man-ch'ing's T'ai Chi Ch'uan.* Berkeley, CA: North Atlantic Books.

Magoun, H. I., Sr. (1976). *Osteopathy in the Cranial Field* (3rd ed.). Kirksville, MO: Journal Printing Company.

Melmed, S., Polonsky, K. S., Larsen, P. R., and Kronenberg, H. M. (Eds.). (2016). *Williams Textbook of Endocrinology* (13th ed.). Philadelphia, PA: Elsevier.

National Center for Health Statistics. (2025). *Multiple cause of death 2018–2023 on CDC WONDER database.* Retrieved February 1, 2025, from https://wonder.cdc.gov/mcd.html

Pine, R. (1996). *Lao-tzu's Taoteching.* San Francisco, CA: Mercury House.

Powers, S. K. (2025). *Diaphragm Function in Health and Disease.* In L. L. Ji (Ed.), The skeletal muscle: Plasticity, degeneration and epigenetics (Vol. 1478). Advances in Experimental Medicine and Biology. Cham, Switzerland: Springer.

Ramraj, B., et al. (2021). *Study on Age of Menarche Between Generations and the Factors Associated With It.* Clinical Epidemiology and Global Health, 11, 100758. https://doi.org/10.1016/j.cegh.2021.100758

Robinet, I. (1997). *The World Upside Down: Essays on Taoist Internal Alchemy.* Albany, NY: State University of New York Press.

Romanes, G. J. (Ed.). (1964). *Cunningham's Textbook of Anatomy* (11th ed.). Oxford, UK: Oxford University Press.

Rosenberg, Z., and Cowan, S. (2025). *A Ring Without End: Reflections on Classical Chinese Medicine Mind/Body Mapping*. San Diego, CA & Cortlandt, NY: Ring Press Collective.

Smith, D. C. (1986). *H. G. Wells: Desperately Mortal*. New Haven, CT: Yale University Press.

Smith, R. W. (1990). *Chinese Boxing, Masters and Methods*. Berkeley, CA: North Atlantic Books.

Song, B. (2024). *Yang Shi's Confucian Quiet-sitting Meditation: A Distinction from Cheng Yi and Huayan Buddhism*. Religions, 15, 1537. https://doi.org/10.3390/rel15121537

Trefts, E., Gannon, M., and Wasserman, D. H. (2017). *The Liver.* Current Biology, 27(21), R1147–R1151. doi:10.1016/j.cub.2017.09.019

Unschuld, P. U. and Hermann, T. 2011. *Huang Di Nei Jing Su Wen: An Annotated Translation of Huang Di's Inner Classic*. Berkley, CA: University of California Press.

Unschuld, P. U. (1988). *Medicine in China: A History of Ideas*. Berkeley, CA: University of California Press.

_____. (2016). *Huang Di Nei Jing Ling Shu: The Ancient Classic on Needle Therapy.* Berkeley, CA: University of California Press.

Wang, A. W., Prieto, J. M., Cauvi, D. M., Bickler, S. W., and De Maio, A. (2020). *The Greater Omentum—A Vibrant and Enigmatic Immunologic Organ Involved in Injury and Infection Resolution.* Shock, *53*(4), 384–390. doi:10.1097/SHK.0000000000001400

Watson, B. (Trans.). (1968). *The Complete Works of Chuang Tzu*. New York, NY: Columbia University Press.

Wells, H. G., Huxley, J., and Wells, G. P. (1939). *The Science of Life*. Garden City, NY: Garden City Publishing Company.

Wilhelm, R. (1931). *The Secret of the Golden Flower: A Chinese Book of Life* (C. F. Baynes, Trans.). New York, NY: Harcourt, Brace & Company.

_____. (1987). *The I Ching or Book of Changes* (C. F. Baynes, Trans.). Princeton, NJ: Princeton University Press.

Wilms, S. (2018). *Humming with Elephants: The Great Treatise on the Resonant Manifestations of Yin and Yang*. Happy Goat Productions.

Wong, E. (2007). *Tales of the Dancing Dragon: Stories of the Tao*. Boston, MA: Shambhala Publications.

Wu, K.M. (1982). *Chuang Tzu: World Philosopher at Play*. New York, NY: Crossroad Publishing Company.

Yang, F. C., Desai, A. B., Esfahani, P., Sokolovskaya, T. V., and Bartlett, D. J. (2021). *Effectiveness of Tai Chi for Health Promotion of Older Adults: A*

Scoping Review of Meta-analyses. American Journal of Lifestyle Medicine, 16(6), 700–716. doi:10.1177/15598276211001222

Yeh, G. Y., Wang, C., Wayne, P. M., and Phillips, R. S. (2008). *The Effect of Tai Chi Exercise on Blood Pressure: A Systematic Review*. Preventive Cardiology, 11(2), 82–89. doi:10.1111/j.1751-7141.2008.07565.x

Zareie, M., Fabbrini, P., Hekking, L. H. P., Keuning, E. D., ter Wee, P. M., Beelen, R. H. J., & van den Born, J. (2006). *Novel role for mast cells in omental tissue remodeling and cell recruitment in experimental peritoneal dialysis*. Journal of the American Society of Nephrology, 17(12), 3447–3457. doi:10.1681/ASN.2005111173

Zhang, J., Niu, C., Ye, L., Huang, H., He, X., Tong, W.-G.,Cheng, T. (2007). *Hematopoietic Stem Cells with Higher Hematopoietic potential Reside at the Bone Marrow Endosteum*. Stem Cells, 25(4), 1062–1069. doi:10.1634/stemcells.2006-0561

About the Author & Translators

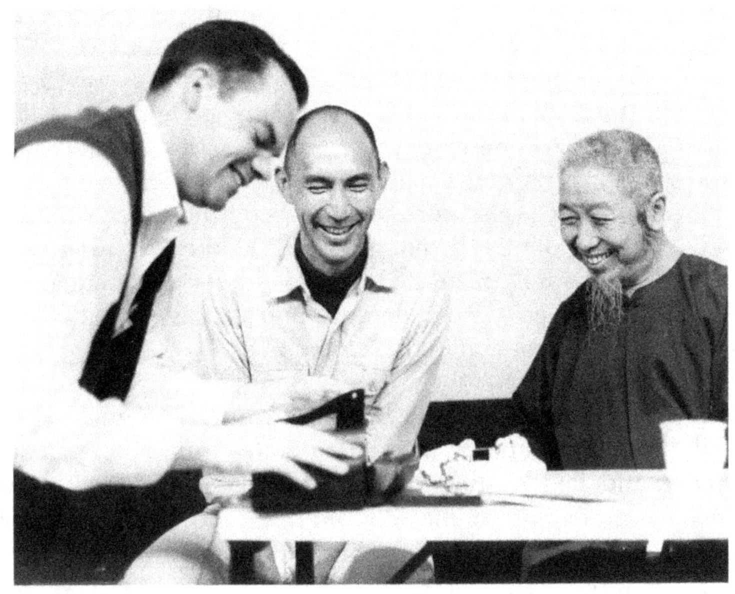

Photo taken around the time Professor Cheng was composing the *Sage Principles*. Image from left to right: Tam Gibbs, Ed Young, and Professor Cheng Man-ch'ing
Photo from Ed Young's Private Collection

Cheng Man-ch'ing (1902-1975) (Author) was a master of *tàijí* 太極 (tai chi), painting, poetry, calligraphy, and Chinese medicine. Born in early 20th-century southeastern China, he showed prodigious talent in the arts from a young age, supporting his family through painting and later teaching poetry and painting at prestigious institutions in Beijing and Shanghai. A leader in China's art world, he also studied Chinese medicine and the classics. After developing Lung disease, he began studying *tàijí* with Yáng Chéngfŭ 楊澄甫, eventually becoming one of the art's most influential teachers while using his medical knowledge to heal and guide others.

Tam Gibbs (1939-1981) (Translator) was a senior American student and trusted associate of Professor Cheng Man-ch'ing during his teaching in 1960s–70s New York City until Professor's death. Serving as secretary, translator and chronicler, Gibbs played a vital role in preserving Cheng's work and legacy, most notably through his English translation of the professor's funerary biography after Cheng's passing in 1975, as well as Professor Cheng's translation of and commentary on the *Dàodé jīng* (*Lao Tzu: My Words Are Very Easy to Understand: Lectures on the Tao Teh Ching* 1981). A prominent teacher in the early development of Professor Cheng's Yang-style *tàijí quán* in America, he appears in archival footage as a senior push hands partner alongside Cheng and fellow student Ed Young. Active at the Shr Jung School, Gibbs was widely respected for his deep understanding of Cheng's shortened Yang-style form and for his lasting contributions to its transmission in the United States.

Ed Young (1931–2023) (Translator), an award-winning children's book illustrator, came to the United States from Shanghai at age twenty and began studying *tàijí* 太極 (Tai Chi) in 1964 with Cheng Man-Ch'ing at the Shr Jung Tai Chi Ch'uan School in New York City. One of Cheng's senior students, Young served as a principal translator and teacher, helping introduce the master's 37-movement Yang-style form to a wider audience. At Cheng's request, he went on to teach in Hastings-on-Hudson, NY for more than forty-five years, bringing the benefits of *tàijí* to generations of students.

Stephen Cowan (Translator), is a western trained pediatrician as well as a Chinese Medical practitioner with 40 years of clinical experience promoting health in children and their families. He is a long-time student of *tàijí quán,* having first studied with C.T. Wu and then for many years with Ed Young, with whom he collaborated on several children's books. He is author of several books on Chinese medicine including *Fire Child, Water Child: How Understanding the Five Types of ADHD Can Help You Improve Your Child's Self-Esteem and Attention (2012)* and *A Ring Without End: Reflections on Classical Chinese Medicine Mind/Body Mapping* (2025).

www.ingramcontent.com/pod-product-compliance
Lightning Source LLC
LaVergne TN
LVHW020708110826
845149LV00012B/2164

* 9 7 9 8 9 9 2 6 8 6 8 2 1 *